Reboot, Reclaim and Refocus Nutrition

Reboot, Reclaim and Refocus Nutrition

A Real Conversation About Energetic and Physical Nutrition

by

Sherry Bainbridge, PhD

Reboot, Reclaim & Refocus Nutrition: A Real Conversation About Energetic and Physical Nutrition

ISBN 978-1-7358688-4-4 (Paperback)
ISBN 978-1-7358688-2-0 (Digital)

NUTRITION / Health & Wellness

Cover and Interior Design: Just Right Productions
Photographer: Susan Estes, Estes Photography

2nd edition, November 2023

Printed in physical and digital form
in the United States of America.

Dedication

I dedicate this book to my sons, Alexander (bless your soul) and Nicholas, who have taken me through many epochs, unexpected lessons and life journeys. Thank you for the gift of four kind-hearted and beautiful grandchildren. There is simply no position more amazing than that of being a mother and grandmother. *I love you!*

Thank you so much for reading this book. I am honored to have put it together to help others understand they are more capable than they realize. People in the world are healing themselves from all sorts of things in spite of secrecy and falseness in the world. If these pages help you better understand and rise above it all, I am deeply grateful.

—Sherry Bainbridge, PhD

Table of Contents

Foreword

In a world that often feels like a whirlwind of chaos, stress and uncertainty, the pursuit of vibrant health and well-being becomes not just a choice but a necessity. It is within this realm of challenges and choices that Sherry Bainbridge invites you to embark on a transformative journey—one that will reboot, reclaim and refocus your understanding of nutrition and its profound impact on your life.

I had the privilege of meeting Sherry under rather serendipitous circumstances in an Uber ride in Denver. I was in town to attend Dr. Joe Dispenza's advanced retreat, seeking deeper insights into the intricacies of the human mind. Little did I know that the Universe had a different plan for that moment, one that would introduce me to a remarkable individual on a mission to empower others with the knowledge and wisdom she had gathered throughout her lifetime.

As an E-RYT (500-hour) yoga instructor, a dedicated Pilates and fitness instructor, and now a student pursuing a double doctorate in Neuroscience and Psychology, my journey has been shaped by my own personal trials and triumphs. I am also a combat veteran, having served in Kosovo. I returned with a life-altering neck injury that, according to medical experts, held the potential to leave me forever paralyzed from the neck down. However, I chose a path that ultimately led me to discover the incredible healing power of breathwork.

My story is just one of countless narratives that illustrate the resilience of the human spirit and the capacity for transformation. It is also a testament to the profound impact that individuals like Sherry Bainbridge can have on our lives. Sherry's book, *Reboot, Reclaim and Refocus Nutrition,* is a beacon of knowledge, insight and hope in a culture too often ensnared by misinformation, deception and corporate interests.

In the pages that follow, Sherry takes you on a journey of discovery—a journey that begins with a candid acknowledgment of the myriad stressors that plague our modern existence. Our society is bombarded by physical, chemical and emotional pressures, and it's no surprise many of us find ourselves trapped in a perpetual state of anxiety. The toll this takes on our immune systems and higher brain functions cannot be overstated. Sherry pulls back the curtain to reveal the powerful forces at play which thrive on our perpetual stress.

Certain mega-wealthy corporations have realized that keeping individuals in a state of perpetual stress can be incredibly profitable. As you delve deeper into this book, you will become acutely aware of the wide-reaching deceptions that shroud the realm of nutritional health. But fear not, for Sherry is here to illuminate the path toward clarity and empowerment.

Throughout her lifetime, Sherry has dedicated herself to helping others gain a profound understanding of how to nourish both body and mind. We are flooded with tummy fillers and mind cloggers, but we have the power to choose what enters our bodies and minds. Armed with the right knowledge, these choices can be simpler than we ever imagined.

The essence of this book can be distilled into a simple yet powerful message: you must be your own detective, your own advocate, in the pursuit of optimal health and well-being. Thriving becomes a daunting challenge within a system designed for the mega-wealthy elite. However, it is a challenge we can overcome, and it begins with a reboot of our understanding, a reclamation of our power and a refocusing of our priorities.

Sherry Bainbridge, PhD, invites you on this life-altering journey with an open heart and a curious mind. With each page you turn, you will gain a deeper appreciation for the profound connection between nutrition and the vitality of your body and mind. You will unearth the tools and insights needed to make informed choices, to distinguish fact from fiction and to empower yourself with the knowledge necessary to thrive in an often bewildering world.

Reboot, Reclaim and Refocus Nutrition is a masterpiece of enlightenment. This guidebook will empower you to take charge of your own health and well-being. It is a testament to the fact that we were all born with the innate capacity to discover the secrets of a vibrant life. As Sherry so eloquently reminds us, "Nutrition is what the body and mind crave the most," and it is within our power to provide it.

In closing, I want to express my deepest gratitude to Sherry for the profound impact she has had on my life and for the countless lives she will touch through this book. It is my sincere hope that you, the reader, will embrace the wisdom contained within these pages and begin your own journey of self-discovery and transformation.

With an open heart and a thirst for knowledge, let us collectively embark on this remarkable voyage that will empower us to reboot, reclaim and refocus our understanding of nutrition. In doing so, we will reclaim the power that resides within each of us.

Leland Holgate, Sr.
The Willful Warrior

Preface

At nine years old, I died and went to the other side. I was given the choice to stay or come back. Coming from a toxic home, they were not sure (and neither was I) if I could fulfill my main purpose for coming here. Obviously, I chose to come back. Nutrition, both energetic and physical, has always been a huge interest and focus of mine.

Living life has left me with injuries from head to toe. I was told I would not be able to function and would likely spend my time on the couch gaining weight. I decided to formally educate myself in Eastern, Tribal and Western healings and spiritual philosophies around the world, using many approaches and modalities. I earned a Masters and PhD in Holistic Health in 2010.

At one point, I was informed by Western medicine that I needed immediate aggressive chemotherapy for a rare bone marrow cancer called *polycythemia vera*. I refused. I wanted to make sure I had it before considering such a radical approach. I put into action every skill, knowledge and technique I could think of to lower the marker. I shocked everyone when a subsequent bone marrow biopsy did not reveal cancer. Western medicine has not discovered anyone else in the world who has done this. It is such a privilege to share with others whatever I can to aid in their healing journey.

My major focus is with past-life regression and dealing with human attachment removal and stop-smoking hypnotherapy. I also offer individualized coaching for holistic and intuitive development. What I do eases struggles and changes lives. It is beautiful and humbling.

This book is packed with information, practical knowledge and techniques to promote true growth with a deeper understanding of how to live and be healthier. If you feel stuck or confused about the world and want to know how you can be healthier, this book is for you.

Acknowledgments

I want to thank my dear friends, Brad Gill, Susan Estes and John Krol for the encouragement, input and support you have provided me along the way. This book could not be possible without you three. I love you all and am so blessed you call me your friend. *Thank you!*

Special author note:

Before doing any health technique or service, please ground yourself by performing the following:

Receptive Healing Technique

Intend for healing and loving energy from the Divine to enter your body through the crown chakra (top center of the head), down through all the chakras, past the root chakra (genitals) and out through your feet into the loving and healing part of earth. Gently bring this healing energy back up through the main chakras and out through your crown into the Universe. This cleans the imbalance from the lower chakras so it does not infect the higher ones and will set the stage for healing.

Introduction

We all come from the same source. There is no need to have a full understanding of it all, nor do we have to agree on the specifics. In the beginning, there was nothing at all. A particle formed and articulated: *LIFE!* Love of life and learning are the basis of this Universe's energy. The Creator/God/Great Spirit/Source/The I am/The All That Is/Yahweh perfected purified love through eons of learning and experiencing. It is a human choice to be committed to growth, loyal to our life purpose and grateful for opportunities that physical and spiritual life provide. This supports the light of love, compassion and kindness.

There are dark things which involve negativity, learning, control, and so forth. The light side of the Universe is about love and learning, and so forth. There are two sides to our world and everything lies in between. Our health is of the utmost importance—more than just physical nutrition, but also energetic nutrition. This feeds our energy and individual growth. Growth is common sense which has become wisdom.

The goal for most on Earth is to become authentic, connected, honest and wise toward the Universe, the Earth, others and ourselves—to rediscover who we really are and rise above that which keeps us blind and limited. We are babies in this Universe! Our focus is to be genuine and see how amazingly capable we are in a world that does much to prevent this from happening. You know the feeling of looking at those in power and wondering *what the heck?* It does not make sense.

To begin this journey, we must give ourselves permission to find value in the authentic self and the self beyond this human experience. If we assume otherwise, we will function under a different belief. We are told, shown and herded by powers who wish to maintain control. They know the power of thought and energy. They are the big companies and corporations that control most everything in our world. They are above government and are large contributors to manipulating the economy and our laws.

The mind is incredible. Miracles can happen when we focus our attention, as in meditation, emotion and awareness. There is no reason for average people to follow unhealthy paths. Disease, illness, sluggishness and disruptive moods all contribute to our experience here. It does not have to be this way for most people. This is a natural process where people catch on and realize there is much more a person can do. Regardless of not having the power and influence of the mega-companies, we do have choice as to what we put into our mouth. One cannot be separated from the other. Everyone is 90% energy. Thoughts are energy, and we need to wrap our heads around the truth of the world we live in.

The truth is that our world is not singular. It represents the Universe as our bodies do. There is life upon life upon life. Much is happening that is hidden from the public. There can be no denying that decisions are being made for profit rather than for health.

The human body requires natural and real food (what comes directly from the earth) and clean hydration to survive. However, laws allow food processors to leave in or add heavy metals, natural and unnatural poisons and fillers, all of which keep processed items full of sugar, fat and salt. These ingredients keep the population sluggish, vulnerable to illness and disease, and deprived of sleep. It is our job to see through this and create change!

We need to let go of what we thought was true and face reality so we can choose better. It's not easy changing what we believe to be true when so much of what we think we know supports those in power and their ultimate goals. They have done a great job of "educating" us to their points of view.

This book is focused on educating you to think differently so you can let go of previous false beliefs and take back your power and choice. This is not just an American issue, but one that affects the world.

Many aboriginals in Australia have had their traditional foods removed and are now forced to consume poisoned food and water. Why would this be allowed to happen? Because it makes people sick and more willing to cooperate.

(Does this ring any bells with what's going on in America today?) Their lands have been undergoing the Americanization of unhealthy flour, rice and sugar. They had a profound connection with their traditional foods which contain physical, energetic and spiritual nutrition. They want *their* nutritious foods, but it's an ongoing fight. Diabetes, heart disease and kidney failure are now affecting the tribes, which has never before been an issue. This is all too common with the non-nutritious processed Western diet.[1]

In the UK, Dr. Chris van Tulleken tested a processed diet for 30 days. He gained 15 pounds and took 10 years off his life. His brain created new connections which increased repetitive eating behavior, very similar to how the brain rewires for tobacco and alcohol addictions. He also suffered negative digestive and other issues that affected his energy, sleep and overall functioning.[2]

Consider the heavy metals in baby food. About every five years, a report comes out stating these concerns, but nothing is done to change anything.[3] Some metals cannot be avoided, but should be removed whenever possible because they are an additional toxin. The body needs to be exposed to build the immune system. However, adding additional stress on a developing brain and body does not make sense. Governments and connected organizations have

1 Annabelle Wilson, Roland Wilson, Robyn Delbridge, Emma Tonkin, Claire Palemo, John Coveney, Colleen Hays, and Tamara Mackean, "Resetting the Narrative in Australian Aboriginal and Torres Strait Islander Nutrition Research," Current Developments in Nutrition, May 18 2020, www.ncbi.nlm.nih.gov > pmc

2 BBC, Dr. Chris van Tulleken, "UK doctor switches to 80% ULTRA-processed food diet for 30 days," September 22, 2021, YouTube: https://youtu.be/T4PFt4czJw0

3 Russell Brand, "You Aren't Going To Like This," September 2022, YouTube: https://youtu.be/5QClLdrbkw8

lied, broken contracts and overlooked much in support of those with money—the real power! Ten companies control nearly everything you buy: Pepsico, Mars, Nestle, Kellogg's, and Associated British Foods are but a few.[4] No country is immune to this. Their billions and trillions of dollars change laws, manipulate the economy, and are the reason governments are not "for the people".

The world has always been this way. Those who have the funds to alter events have influence on the outcome. They can direct money in a controlled and consistent way. This is how business works. The Rockefellers were involved in American medical education while their petroleum products were simultaneously aiding pharmaceutical development.[5] They contributed to many schools while demanding that natural healing was not to be part of the curriculum.

As an individual, I want healing—not just symptom relief. Integrity is a casualty of profit. We must take responsibility for our health or suffer the consequences of ill health. Choosing health is depicted as difficult and is made to be confusing. My goal is to clear out some of the confusion and to make nourishment easier to understand as a part of life. It is a lifestyle.

All my life I have had an interest in health. I watched my obese parents suffer with self-image, illness and disease. They bought into every fad diet. When frozen dinners came out, my mother was so elated that she stacked our grocery cart

---

4 Lindsay Mattison, "10 of the Biggest Food Companies Basically Own Every Grocery Item You Buy," May 3 2022, www.wideopeneats.com/biggest-food-companies/

5 Meridian Health Clinic, "How Rockefeller Created the Business of Western Medicine," December 27 2019, How Rockefeller Created the Business of Western Medicine – Acupuncture & Dry Needling, Santa Monica, CA (meridianhealthclinic.com)

with them. High fat, sugary and salty items—they bought cases and cases of diet soda and thought nothing of drinking many cans in one day. I still see people buying these foods in my grocery store today.

As a child, I was appalled. It was obvious to me what was causing their health issues. They wanted a quick fix and did not want to face what they did not want to change. Thinking attracts like energy. Becoming adaptable with thinking is a huge breakthrough.

Leaving home at 17 was a challenge. Shortly thereafter, I lost my job. This was a serious situation because jobs were hard to come by. I lucked out and got a job as a food runner at a nearby restaurant. I made sure the orders were what the customers wanted, and I garnished the plates before the waitresses took them out. The owners were very kind to me. I lived on cheesecake, shrimp, Beef Wellington, quality fish and salads; and they never once complained. They knew I was literally starving. Many of the waitresses were models. I had never seen a person grab a leaf of lettuce and eat it straight. They taught me that we really do have choice, and so much more. This was the start of my healthier food awareness.

This book is a lifetime of information, formal and self-education, and thousands upon thousands of hours of research. Many times, I have had to change what I thought was true.

A majority of people have acquired the opinions of others and have never done the work to discover things for themselves. I get it. Life can get really busy. Information is confusing and contradictive. There's no doubt the information in these pages will change over time; but for now, it gives a real and concise look at what we can do to create a healthy and vibrant life!

Human life demands a moment-by-moment choice: recognizing the truth or living by the opinions of others. In the midst of adjusting to and living with purpose and becoming someone we can truly love, be kind to and deeply care about, we can learn to love and care for others. This is not selfishness; rather, it is a means to maintaining a healthy mental, physical, spiritual and energetic frequency. Practicing on ourselves helps heal us and prepare us for loving others.

Understanding who we are amid selfish and contrary agendas is certainly a challenge. This is nothing new. Remember in elementary school when the teacher sat everyone in a circle? She whispered a short sentence to the first student, then that student repeated it. By the time it came back around the circle, there was NO resemblance to the original sentence. It does not take much to fool and distract people. We are far more controllable, predictable and able to be influenced when disconnected from our divine energetic core. This part of us contains information that can affect what we accomplish in this life. It raises and lowers vibration based on what we are believing. It affects every aspect of life.

Like the earth, our body is a sensitive communication resource center that is designed to support us. It tells us what it needs and when it needs it. If a person ignores the body's communication, it will speak louder and try to educate us; yet it continues to support the thinking we are choosing. There is no separation from the Universe, from each other or from ourselves. Ultimately, everything has been created from that original source. This is why we are all connected. We are each different, yes; but are nevertheless related to all creation.

Remember the American government constantly denying its remote viewing program? Remote viewing is the ability to see and describe a distant place, person, lifeform, etc. The government and its agencies used a developed process in which a viewing team would draw an unknown location leaders wanted to know more about. Some initiatives can envision without drawing, but the methods they used also worked. For 35 years, government agencies and corporations used intuitive individuals to train and develop their programs. Physicists then discovered a scientific aspect to remote viewing. Physicist and parapsychologist, Russell Targ, speaks very openly about this.[6]

I spent a day speaking with author Angela Thompson Smith, PhD, who was involved in the program for 35 years. She wrote several books on the subject.[7] [8] [9] Other great books are *The Essential Guide to Remote Viewing,* by Paul H. Smith, PhD, and *Remote Viewing Dialogues,* by Daz Smith (a psychic spy veteran of 23 years with US military Intelligence). When I returned home, I attempted remote viewing. This single experience was easy. It is just another means of

---

6 Russell Targ, "Russell Targ physicist on Telepath, Remote Viewing Banned TED talk, April 16, 2019, YouTube: https://youtu.be/FI_01m-6L30

7 Angela Thompson Smith PhD, "Remote Perceptions," July 2016, Triangular Publishing

8 Angela Thompson Smith PhD, "Seer", 2016, Triangular Publishing

9 C.B. Scott Jones Ph.D. and Angela T. Smith Ph.D., "Voices From the Cosmos," 2014, Headline Books

accessing information and knowledge in the energetic field. Science has proven it!

We earthly humans are like infants in the way we comprehend all of this. This is why the mind must have time to evolve and develop before moving to the next level. Learning stretches our brain by rewiring and reconnecting it. It's uncomfortable and is rarely an easy process. This is easier than you might believe, but please keep reading and try to embrace it. Have you ever taken a class and felt very confused, but by the end it all just came together and made sense? Stay on course. Knowledge is power! Even healthy, natural food has glitches we should know about. Lighten up. It's fun and enriching to have a good handle on the many nutritional choices available.

Unfortunately, we also need a good understanding of why we are so confused. We need to stop believing in our own inabilities to determine truth. This makes us vulnerable to manipulations in being told what, when, how, or even whether to think, feel and act. The world has always been this way. It is nothing new. Focus on power based on a many a dollar. Here is how I think the formula looks:

The Secure Profitability Formula

Consistent + Predictable + Controllable Profits =
Secure profits from this time forward

This formula rules the earth! Complain all we want, but most people are not the ones in power. Much research and effort has gone into determining how to maintain and enhance this formula's outcome. As costs continue to rise, so do the efforts to influence where the food and beverage dollars go. This practice has gone to the extreme using so many different schemes that it's highly confusing to figure out what is healthy and what is not. Weeding through all the studies is mindboggling because they contradict each other's findings. It's ever-changing and altering in order to keep us confused and to maintain control as things evolve. Large and small business can lack integrity by taking things too far. This is not a surprise. There will always be a point in time where the pendulum swings back in the other direction because something has gone too far. Then more people get knowledgeable and determined enough to take action by embracing healthy, energetic and physical nutrition.

Changes easily go unnoticed, such as label requirements changing in 2016. Edible products now have serving sizes which are double the size from years ago. Many people will consume the larger serving size without noticing. When calories *from* fat are replaced with the *type* of fat, it can be confusing. Trans, saturated, mono-unsaturated and polyunsaturated fats are indistinguishable for most people. Added sugars are now required (even those in processing), but can be overlooked with so many different names for sugars. Honey, maple syrup and a bag of sugar have different labeling requirements. Multiple sugar ingredients with over 30 different names such as corn sweetener, ethyl maltol, corn of any kind, and fructose[10] are required on the label as of 2018.[11] The lower on the ingredients list, the less percent-

10 Admin at Total Health Chiropractic Blog, "30 Names for Hidden Sugars!," July 31 2020, https://totalhealthhixson.com/blog/30-names-for-hidden-sugars/

11 US Office of the President UCLA Newsroom, "No more sneaking sugar into packaged

age of that item is in a product. Higher up on the list indicates a larger amount. However, just because an ingredient shows up lower does not mean there is less of it. Many people choose to simply look at an ingredient's position on the list. When added up, though, it can be shocking to see just how much sugar there really is. Many protein bar labels are excellent examples. These can contain many different sugars in small amounts, adding up to very high amounts of sugar.

Health verbiage should generally be ignored, such as natural, healthy, low-fat, diet or light.[12] Just being low in fat and calories is not enough. The product should be low in sugar and flour products and be nutritious. Labels are also inconsistent. Vitamin D requirements are on the label, but Vitamins A and C are not required (www.fda.gov/food).

If a product contains raspberry flavoring, there is no requirement to include the ingredients of the flavoring or any enhancing ingredients, such as flavonoids. An online search could very well reveal beaver or pig butt oil. Company responses on these types of ingredients are vague and give only a semblance of an answer. Food processors and controllers are very good at making labeling difficult to understand. Many games are played to hide the truth and to make light of the truth. Hidden ingredients are designed to cause specific and intense flavor on the tongue or to make it taste more realistic. It is common that raspberry flavoring is not from raspberries at all. Often, it is chemically derived.

---

foods," June 30 2016, https://newsroom.ucla.edu/stories/no-more-sneaking-sugar-into-packaged-foods

12 Helen West, RD with Healthline, "8 Ways Food Companies Hide the Sugar Content of Foods," April 9 2019, #6, https://www.healthline.com/nutrition/8-ways-sugar-is-hidden#TOC_TITLE_HDR_7

Carboplunks are designed with chemicals to cause flavor to be wonderful, but it disappears in moments. In this way, you are unable to savor and truly enjoy the food. The goal is to cause a person to desire more because it leaves one unsatisfied on energetic and physical levels. Nutritious and real quality items have flavors that linger so they can be appreciated, but artificial formulas undermine such pleasure. Did you know the percentage of daily value on labels are based on the serving size and on how many nutrients it contains for the recommended amount for a person aged 4 and older? The percentages are misleading! Real, healthy food contains what the body needs to be nourished. Even so, healthy foods contain their own natural hazards which are not listed on labels.

Metals and unnatural poisons are not included on the label. The government has limits on how much a product can contain, but they do not usually enforce their own rules. Incidences of overweight, diabetes, cancers and food allergies (among others) are continually rising. Health is deteriorating, not increasing.

Profitable agendas pull us in many directions and cause great confusion, distrust and misdirection. It muddles the mind. It's no wonder people throw up their hands and avoid the whole mess, but this response has shown to be costly to mental and physical health. We must rise above and learn to listen to what our bodies have to say. If you get gassy after eating an item, feel bloated or nauseous, get a rash, start itching, have an accumulation of mucus in the throat or have a foggy head, it's the body's way of telling you that the food you ate is *not* what it needs or wants.

Each physical body is unique; there is no one-size-fits-all formula. Therefore, each person must learn to listen carefully and assist the body so it can be supportive with health and well-being. There are many licensed and alternative professionals who can test for allergies and sensitivities. Keep in mind, though, that some people may not test positive, even if they are. Kinesiology, hypnotherapy and many other approaches can really help hone in on what your body needs and wants.

If you owned a restaurant and discovered that the colors orange, yellow and red have vibrational properties which increase appetite, wouldn't you likely paint the walls with one of these colors and avoid other color frequencies which limit hunger? Keep in mind that those involved in schemes also have families to care for, others to answer to, and desire to hold onto what they have. Our negative judgment of them is not helpful, but our actions in choosing what to spend our money on is important. Money talks.

The more authentic a person becomes, the less likely they will be influenced. The world continues to discredit and discourage such self-development and freethinking, as it undermines the formula.

Stress is the leading cause of illness. In fact, 90% of all illness is stress related.[13] Stress is defined as a process in which environmental demands can strain an organism's adaptive capacity, resulting in both psychological demands and bio-

13 Clemson University Cooperative Extension Service, Lesson 1 revised by Brenda J. Thames EdD and Deborah J. Thomason, EdD, "Stress Management for the Health of It," February 1997,

logical changes that could place one at risk for illness.[14] Stress is caused by the mind! 9.99% of ailment is toxin related, and that tiny .01% is a natural pathogen[15] (a bacterium, virus, or other microorganism that cause disease). This book initially focuses on how a person thinks and attempts to help people align their thinking in such a way that it benefits life. Healthy thinking aligns us with important feelings and is absolutely a superpower. Take control of your own thinking, stop running from it and don't give it away. Don't let others rule your mind, lives and relationships!

Notice the words you speak and think. Each word has its own vibration, a frequency of energy. These are highly potent. Their powerful effects (proven in science) either enhance, stagnate or sabotage. For the purpose of this book, let's drop the word *FOOD* and replace it with *NUTRITION* or *NOURISHMENT!* The definition of food has become so muddled that people believe fake food is real food. The body needs both energetic and physical nourishment to be at its best and to have the strength to overcome when not at its peak. Words have intense power. They align the mind, body and spirit. They support each of them and their underlying meanings.

Words support attitudes and beliefs, which then cause actions and reactions that support them. Use words carefully and wisely. If I say that I wish for more money, I'm really

---

14 Cohen S, Kesslet RC, Gordon LU, "Strategies for measuring stress in studies of psychiatric and physical disorders," Measuring stress: A guide for Health and Social Scientists, Oxford University Press; 1995, Cohen: Measuring stress: A guide for health and social... - Google Scholar

15 Dr. Joe Dispenza, stated in "Heal" Documentary, 2017, https://www.healdocumentary.com/purchase.html (as well as, many other places for purchase or rent)

saying I fear not having enough. However, if I give thanks for money, it comes easy to me. Then I let go of the thought and trust energy to take over, while simultaneously putting forth balanced and healthy actions that bring in money. The physical and spiritual can now provide support where needed. Notice and modify the words you think and use. Make them gentle, truthful and real. Don't exaggerate. Don't criticize yourself for every word that pops in your head, as there are many influences. Just be aware of their power and participate with them so they can increase the good. This is a form of helpful manipulation. Find real, honest and humble ways to make it work.

If one word is not working or does not align with your goals, replace it with one that does. I don't mean to make stuff up through words. Notice the words and let them clue you in to ways of thinking that aren't working. Choose words that are gentle, forgiving, inspiring and truthfully supportive. Words are literal and matter-of-fact. There's no reason we can't healthfully condition our own thinking so that it becomes more effective. You are in control and can create your own results toward healthier actions, reactions and words. This will provide the needed foundation for the body, mind and spirit to be positively supportive. The body and spirit will step up to the emotional and physical plate we feed them every single time.

Everyone knows someone who thinks the way they see the world is absolutely accurate, even when facts contradict them. Many learn to be unwavering and narrow-minded in their thinking. Life was designed to grow and expand thinking. The brain is not meant to be on autopilot. When this happens, it can overcompensate for feeling insecure or not being seen as smart enough. This can give a person a false sense of feeling better than others. When someone thinks in this manner, physical changes within the brain foster an inability to think otherwise. The brain bypasses the section that is no longer being used. As time goes on, it becomes harder, more challenging, and nearly impossible to think differently. Narcissists (those selfish all-about-me people), fanatics and addicts are great examples. This is a proven energetic brain phenomenon. If you tell your brain that you don't need it, it will shut down! All life forms are meant to explore and to keep learning so the brain stays active. There are many books out there which are based on research that shows the impressive ability to rewire and reignite stagnant and sleeping parts of the brain. However, when the brain is damaged or if cells get killed off (as through heavy drug addiction), it becomes much harder and will take longer; but it's not impossible.

There are many ways to exercise the brain. In fact, it is my belief that we are here to solve problems. It's not a comfortable process when we experience or learn something challenging. It stretches the brain because it is meant to. Be kind to yourself and don't give up.

Keep learning different approaches and different ways of thinking. Notice when discomfort arises and ask yourself what the underlying thinking may be. If rooted in a negative idea or one that is not inclusive, caring, kind, loving, and gentle, then face it, explore it and dig deep to find and correct it. It always leads to better clarity about yourself and life. It's not a threat to know the truth. The truth sets people free, right?

Natives and successful tribes around the world are adaptable through their thinking. They are more realistic about their coexistence (human is not the only human-like species) here on Earth and have incredible knowledge about the cosmos. They are not void of corruption in their beliefs, as all have their own truths and non-truths; but I believe they have more facts than other groups around the world. Truth has always been highly regarded in most all tribes around the world. It's so significant that lying could get you kicked out or murdered. Their treasured history is the most accurate around. It's worth studying in more depth if you wish to know more truths about this multi-existent world.

It is impossible to ignore how bombarded society is with negative messages of shaming, guilt and blame. This is not of our creator, but of humans and others who support the formula. It is meant to put people in fear. "…the best way to control a populace is through fear and discord."[16] Fear produces cooperation and stagnation, and invites the same energy. Whether tangible, intangible, real or imagined, it has been used as a means of blackmail, punishment, manipulation, conditioning, sales, fear of judgment, being different, not being enough, death, health and so on. Fear has been used to manipulate people and to block clear thinking. When in fear, hormones rage, defensiveness rises, fight or flight sets in, and thinking can become very scrambled. People are

---

16 John Whitehead of Daily Progress, "Fear is being used to manipulate the public," December 27 2015, https://dailyprogress.com/fear-is-being-used-to-manipulate-the-public/article_3b5d0cc5-3a13-5b4a-a251-0826a7d12140.html

taught to stop, drop and roll if they catch fire. This saying is practiced over and over. Why? Because the initial reaction (flight) is to run from danger, which only inflames the fire. Fear undermines truth and wisdom, reducing self-reliance and the ability to determine truth for ourselves. Being able to discern truth involves confirmation, energy and spirit guidance. Many ancient writings state to not trust the eyes and ears, as they can easily be deceived. But energy cannot be so easily deceived if a person is in tune to its skillful ability to communicate guidance. It is as Aristotle said: "He who overcomes his fears will truly be free."

Let go of unhealthy fears. If being chased by a lion, this would be a healthy fear. Let go of unhealthy ones, which are not real but created so that people will follow others and spend money with little or no questions asked.

Knowledge can be used to influence others and become a tool of intentional manipulation. Notice the repetitiveness of a single line in a catchy tune, as well as in ads, gestures, symbols and slogans. The use of repetitiveness, frequency and vibration is not foreign to those in control. They all use color, hypnosis, meditations, mind control, prayer, light, information, smell, sound, subliminal messages, tastes, words, vibration, visuals and whatever else they need to bring about a desired emotion, thinking and reaction. These are pounded into a person, and over time they will create thinking and behaviors that are not helpful. Tell yourself or others enough times that they are lousy, and eventually they will begin to believe without reason. Thought is the most compelling, effective and active force!

Two dental specialists, one in 1975 and another in 2005,

asked me if I thought I could grow bone. To each one I responded yes. Both professionals admitted that if people did not believe this was possible they would not waste their time explaining it. I grew bone in my cheek (1975) and in a much more difficult area above my upper incisors (2005) in preparation for necessary teeth implants.

When someone with multiple personality or dissociative identity disorder switches identity, the eye color may change. A disease present within one may not be present in the other. One may even speak a different language unknown to a previous personality. What changed in those instances? The thinking changed. Thought is incredibly powerful!

Intentional and unintentional confusions dim and dumb down our connections to internal guidance when we attend to the real self and body. They cause anxiety, disconnection, fear, body abuse, insecurities and laziness. The more these confusions impact the self-image, the more a person spirals down and reaches for external comforts that can never satisfy the appetite. It is an emotional addiction attached to a false solution that only creates more emotional addiction. The strongest hunger is for a real and truthful connection. When truly connected to this amazing energetic and physical body, it is like your very own baby to care for. It deserves nourishing at every level.

When our beingness is valued, we are more likely to treat ourselves and others with greater respect. We are all beautiful, amazing, ordinary human beings with a body within an energy body. Our bodies deserve love, protection and proper nutrition.

In the following pages, I will share the things I focus on

when it comes to what I put into my mouth. This was compiled because I (like so many of my friends and clients) was sick and tired of trying to figure out how to eat healthier. For me, this needed to be clearly laid out and simplified so it would be sustainable over time. It has worked so well that for years I have given this information to hundreds of clients as part of a plan toward better health. You decide what works for you and what will not. Your body and spirit will speak up and be the guide. In the next chapter, I will share a few fun and fascinating techniques to help you understand what your body is saying about what it wants and does not want.

If you treat the body with compassion, love, respect and proper nutrition, it will be less hungry, require less food and be more capable of supporting you in this thinking. It is a choice and a way of life. Change is inevitable. It teaches us to be flexible and adaptable.

If the thinking is not working, the thinking must change. Nothing changes if it stays the same. Stop handing yourself over to outside influencers. In a world where it seems we have few real choices, we *can* choose what we put into our mouths. It's something to be embraced and to get excited about!

After two car accidents, a work accident, an injury from an individual and basic overuse, my body has developed so many structural issues that life and daily exercise are both challenging. I spent 16+ years in formal and self-education within Eastern, Tribal and Western healing and spiritual philosophies. Although I was laid up, I forced myself to take on clients. Their input and successes were amazing. Nothing can be done without the help of others.

In 2007, I pushed the scales above 184 pounds. It demonstrated my life struggles and unhappiness. It's very easy for me to gain weight with obesity and diabetes in my genetics. When I used the information in these pages, I began to lose and maintain my weight. There are many things that must be done to increase health. One approach will ever be enough. I use very little, if any, medication. I shocked Western doctors when I lowered a life-threatening health marker. They were not aware of anyone else in the world doing this. What's in this book really works!

I hope these techniques and views are of value as you determine your best course. I wish no ill will toward anyone nor to any industry; but if something harms instead of helps, then change needs to be made. Let go of the fear of change. Face it with enthusiasm; it is such a gift. I sincerely hope this book will give you the information you've been hungering for. I hope it will aid in a happier, more loving, trusting and deeper relationship with yourself and nutrition. This is all done for the magical and magnificent physical body. So... Reboot, Reclaim and Refocus nutrition so it works for you!

Disclaimer.

Never stop taking prescribed medications without your professional licensed medical team's input. Inform them of any significant life changes. As health increases, a person may be able to lessen, if not eliminate, certain pharmaceuticals at the advice of trusted professionals. Their knowledge and access to technology can be most helpful in tracking and validating health efforts. This book is never to be construed as licensed medical advice or diagnoses. If your medical team is not open-minded in the use of alternative philosophies, search out a team that is. You are worth the effort! We need you, and humanity is not complete without you.

Personal note.

Many perspectives have shaped the views within these pages. Every effort has been made to provide accurate and truthful information. The Reboot, Reclaim and Refocus practice is a customizable plan that will take some time to design. There is no reason to do everything or to go overboard. Be healthfully flexible, have patience, and let your body be the guide.

Above all, *get excited!* This knowledge can help with achieving and maintaining a healthy weight and realizing an improvement in overall health. It enhances the immune system and is highly adaptable. These are the qualities necessary for making lifestyle changes that are livable and will stick.

Life is tough. Please realize that when a person makes life changes they don't often run these by people around them. Change causes reactions, and sometimes people may not realize they tend to pull others back to old familiar behaviors. Be kind, have compassion and change yourself—not others. In time, they will be more accepting of the new you. If not, life still moves forward.

You are DIVINE, WORTH IT, and ENOUGH! Regardless of the life you've chosen, step up, participate, keep learning and healing; and watch life become healthier, more joyful and downright enchanting.

Divine Love and Health,
Sherry

1| Reboot a Desire for Health

We all have ways of sabotaging health and get a lot of outside help to do so. Ever wonder why healthy carbohydrates (fruits, vegetables, and maybe a little grain) are combined with unhealthy ones full of fat, salt and sugar? This is not by accident, and certainly accomplishes the goal of making things confusing. *Reboot, Reclaim and Refocus Nutrition* resolves, at least in part, this confusion by separating healthy and unhealthy carbohydrates.

Healthy Carbohydrates (Benefits) = **Carbohydrates**

- Healthy: fruits and vegetables
- Some health benefits: beans, grains and questionable dairy

We will discuss these in more detail later in this book.

Unhealthy Carbohydrates (Nutrient Starved Tummy Fillers) = ***Carboplunks***

- Salty, fatty and/or sugary items
- Flour based items

- Little to no nutritional value
- Processed or prepared
- Not directly or naturally from the earth
- Genetically modified organisms (GMOs)

People often plunk unhealthy food into the stomach. This makes them feel full and comfortable, and it relieves boredom. These foods, which contain combinations of toxins, chemicals, colorings, flavorings, flavonoids, high salt, high sugar and feed corn to name a few, numb the taste buds and create addiction. The body does not naturally crave these types of foods. The body naturally craves healthy, nutritious and life-supporting items.

Stop internalizing the beliefs you are fed about *carbo-plunks*. Don't beat yourself up with excuses like these: *Everything put in the mouth is either tasteless or going to make you fat anyway; There's no time, so jump in the fast food line; Healthy food takes too much time to prepare;* or, *No one has control over any input for change.* You are in control of your body and mind. Lighten up about yourself because you did not reach this point on your own. The same tactics used to guide you into unhealthy thinking and purchasing can be used by you to increase healthy thinking and purchasing. It just takes a bit of knowledge, changing your thinking, and intentional action on your part.

Things are purposely designed to be confusing and influential, so much that people surrender their choice and settle for what does not make sense. Most of those who are "in the know" are connected to powerful companies and individuals with a great deal of money. They are able to hire chefs to do all the healthy preparation and cooking for them. For them, nearly everything is made from scratch, purchased from local farms, ranches and health food stores; and the majority rarely (if ever) eat *carboplunks*. They must take care of their bodies in order to maintain their lives and businesses. Notice how those few seen in public are usually healthy, not overweight and are physically and mentally active. They have a double standard—different rules for themselves than for the majority of the population that supports their financial success. It's real, and it's a fact. They have their own families, lifestyle and *power*. They don't want to give it up. Would you? Of course not. Set aside preconceived judgment and take on the challenge to do things differently. Don't be a follower without knowledge. Be excited to take control, and take charge of your beliefs!

There is no question how powerful the mind can be in relieving symptoms and healing the body. For example, if you choose to believe that what you're eating is going to end up as fat,[1] it will! This does not mean you should eat crappy foods and expect to not have crappy results just by thinking about it. There are unavoidable physical limitations. Body wisdom is knowing that the body is provided essential nutrition, correct thinking, movement and spiritual balance. Energy has rules, but not the same type as with the physical. Thought is energy, and anything that contains energy has thought. Everything starts with a thought. Thinking is your most powerful tool. Stop handing it over and start using the same knowledge to your advantage!

---

1 Institute for the Psychology of Eating, "Can Thoughts Be Fattening?", approximately 2012, https://psychologyofeating.com/can-thoughts-be-fattening-video-with-emily-rosen/

Reboot thinking.

Thinking has been so controlled and influenced by others that most of us have no idea what the process is to retain common sense, to see the truth through all the hype, and to regain wisdom. There is a process to healing our thinking:

When one thought is changed, it cascades through other existing thoughts, comparing itself to each one. When it encounters an incompatible thought, it generates a negative and conflicting emotion within you. You must analyze the thought behind the emotion and define it. Perceive it honestly and ask, *Why this thought?* Find ways to regard it in a more positive, loving, forgiving and supportive way. Now you have another new thought! This new thought, along with the previous thought, moves throughout the brain and locates older and more incompatible thoughts. As they multiply, each must be acknowledged and modified so that the new thought can continue to assess where other thinking must change.

Negative emotions are divine communications that draw attention to thoughts which do not serve you. The process repeats over and over. It may sound confusing and overwhelming as old thoughts increase in numbers and test your thinking. Don't give up. It gets easier with experience and clears out so many unnecessary and undermining thoughts. There's no reason to argue with it; just keep at it, as with any new subject you learn. This is a process which rewires the brain and ignites the parts that have shut down due to unhealthy thinking. It is not a comfortable process. Learning is usually a bit distressing because it stretches and alters the brain. Embrace this and do not fight it. You experienced the same sensations and feelings learning a new subject in school. It just *is*. Eventually, thinking becomes greater and more easily flexible and adaptable. This is a skill that all advancing humans must develop. Don't give up!

What we've described is often called the process of aligning, and it's how we reboot our thinking. People frequently give up here, but please don't! If you get stuck and can't determine what a thought or emotion means, seek out one or more licensed therapists. There are also alternative approaches, such as acupuncture, coaching, educating, energy work, hypnotherapy, intuitive healing readings, meditations, prayer and tapping. These can be helpful in streamlining the discovery process, which can bring to light any buried and denied experiences tied to the emotions and development of damaged thinking. People are masters at covering up and denying.

Ever work for somebody who treats someone else's mistake like it's the end of the world, and whose threats of firing people are ever looming? It sucks, so don't do it to yourself. Laugh a lot and be kind to yourself!

Here on Earth, we are in school. It's a classroom, a grade to work through—nothing more. Fear of failure, punishment or judgment have little if any value here. Strive for excellence, not perfection. Carefully examine anything you resist. More often than not, it's exactly what you should be doing and overcoming. Each time you face such resistance and get beyond whatever is behind it, you grow. There is a saying: "If you fall off a horse, get right back on." This has great truth. You may need to back off a bit, but keep trying until you can get back on with ease and move forward.

Organize and outline your mind every morning so that you are focused on supporting the outline. At the beginning of the day, set your mind to eat healthily and refuse any thought to the contrary. Thus, the decision is made and arguing is not a choice. The body and mind need nutrition and exercise to properly function and to feel good. If you know that you tend to eat *carboplunks* because the day is busy and you're out and about, throw together something small like an apple or orange, or bag a few prunes along with some healthy nuts to carry with you. Now you have a choice to support the day's healthy goals when the body says it needs nutrition. Keep finding ways to get rid of excuses. Don't allow your thinking to accept an excuse. Keep solving the problems that block you from health. The more you do this, the more obvious excuses will become and the easier it will be to solve them.

The body, like the brain, has its own ability to think. Every single cell has energy and thought. The body knows *when* to do, *how* to do, *what* to do and *if* to do; but it gets confused when thinking is not aligned in healthy ways. Science has proven that anger can changes every cell in the body.[2] The brain itself doesn't change the cells; rather, the cells alter themselves to the flood of thoughts and chemicals the brain sends out. Cells, muscles, organs and body systems either strengthen or weaken according to our thinking. Each cell has memory in which cell or muscle memory[3] is relied

---

2 Louise B. Miller Ph.D., "What Causes Anger and How It Affects the Body," July 16, 2020, https://www.psychologytoday.com/us/blog/the-mind-body-connection/202007/what-causes-anger-and-how-it-affects-the-body

3 Michael Mathews and Scientifically Reviewed by Dr. Brian Grant, "Is Muscle Memory

upon for peak performance, as proven in sports. The athlete practices and practices so they can clear all thinking and stay present with the basics when it's time to perform. The body and cells remember what to do and how to do it. Every athlete knows this. You can aid or undermine your body through your thinking.

Thoughts have frequencies and vibration.[4] In fact, each word has measurable amplification (loudness), frequency (vibrational wavelengths) and vibrations (moving back and forth or side to side). When *speaking* a word, the throat vibrates to make the sound. When *thinking* a word, the brain uses electrical waves and neurons to communicate it.[5] Choose words carefully and disregard those that do not align with your goals. Your thoughts are created and influenced into your mind.[6]

Everything is of Source, and that means you! If you think *idiot*, which people likely do at some point, then immediately reject it! *Not idiot!* Negative words have long-lasting and harmful effects on the mind, body and energy.[7] Words

---

Real? An Answer According to Science," approximately 2012, Blog-Building Muscle at httpslegionathletics.com/muscle-memory/

4 Dr. Kim & Dr. Hil, "The Quantum Mechanics of Changing Thoughts," November 14, 2010, https://www.authenticityassociates.com/the-quantum-mechanics-of-changing-thoughts/

5 Andrea Moro, "Why you can 'hear' words inside your head;" "When we have conscious thoughts, we can often hear a voice inside our heads-now new research is revealing why," September 29 2020, MIT Press Reader, https://www.bbc.com/future/article/20200929-what-your-thoughts-sound-like

6 Eldon Taylor, "Thinking Without Thinking: Who's In Control Of Your Mind?," 1995, Progressive Awareness Research, https://www.progressiveawareness.org/articles/Thinking_Without_Thinking.html

7 Jennifer Gunner, "Effects of negative Words: Common Expressions and Their Power," 2022 , Your Dictionary – Love To Know Media, https://grammar.yourdictionary.com/style-and-usage/affects-of-negative-words.html

are behind every attitude, behavior and action. They are the foundation that determines success or an opportunity (not failure!) to learn.

The fastest way to sabotage positive healthy efforts is by being over-enthusiastic—starting with a plan that is not maintainable over time. Many fad diets have made megabucks on quick weight loss programs that are not doable over the long run. Even professionals have encouraged losing a large amount of weight quickly as an incentive for losing more. The intentions are good, but these actions often set a person up for failure. There is not a one-size-fits-all method. Everyone is different in many ways, and this must be considered when designing your unique healing plan.

The body is here to serve you. It will do so based on your thinking. (Is this sinking in?) Thinking determines actions and reactions. Do you see any patterns connecting this concept in your life? If your thinking can change, all else falls into place in a way that aids rather than destroys.

Professionals often work with clients and patients to discover underlying thinking and use techniques to aid people in changing stuck thinking. One form is visualization, where imagination is used to replace an unwanted reaction rooted in a past experience, even if that thought has been healed. Visualization is a technique that can unstick an experience and replace it with a healthier one. Every time I was around my mother, the memories of her abuse and of my disappointed expectations would rise up and cause unwanted anger and defensiveness. Visualizing is similar to daydreaming. The imagination takes over whether you see it clearly or not. I see clouds with a beautiful blue sky. I leap from one to the other, flying on them and seeing the world. My mind sees the clouds even though my eyes do not. If I asked you to picture a crayon, you may see the words and picture the crayon. This is visualization; it is how we communicate with the subconscious mind. The mind, body and spirit are on the same page. It is a type of reset. In this case, I am resetting my reaction to my mother. It opens legitimate avenues of healing myself, not her. I developed compassion and understanding for her traumas, but my mind was stuck in the reactions, anyway.

I performed this visualization exercise: *I came home from elementary school. My mother greeted me at the door with a big smile and she welcomed me with a great hug. She was happy, joyful and at peace. We walked to the dining table where a homemade snack awaited. As I nibbled the healthy snack, I shared my day with her. She was happy for my day and comforted me around my struggles. She listened and asked a question or two, taking interest in what I had learned.*

This simple exercise gave my mind something positive to draw upon when around my mother. She was a good person with a good heart, but raising children was not something she understood, and her own unresolved wounds came out in highly abusive manners. With something positive for my brain to draw upon, I no longer had a negative or defensive reaction when around her. I would repeat this visualization technique many times until the wise brain drew from the new vision rather than the old. This was part of my healing. It's an amazingly simple, yet powerful, exercise. It has only to do with my thinking. People can often change themselves but not others, so using this technique with someone who has not changed is incredibly helpful. Sometimes, people must walk away from a difficult relationship; but I honestly believe that when a person can adjust to it without getting too involved, it can create growth at every level. This aids in personal evolvement and in a variety of similar situations that may arise in the future. It is a form of self-preservation and adapting to the reality of the relationship.

As a child, I chose to stand up to the abuse and was in my parents faces about it, sharing it with teachers, church members and anyone who would listen. I'm grateful to have been so bold, but these choices left me with my own wounds from which to heal. There is always a price to pay for such ongoing anger and resentfulness.

Facing inconvenient truths about ourselves (and each other) is simply part of a healthy life path. The body knows what it wants and what it does not. Each person must know his or her own body and act on communicating with it. The more the body realizes we are listening and acting upon it, the clearer its communications. It takes awareness, acceptance, flexibility, creativity, a willingness to act on the truth, and an ability to set aside unsupportive thinking in exchange for thinking that supports us—especially when based in love, compassion, kindness and acceptance of differences.

It is seriously important to show the body that you are listening and willing to change. Like all living creatures, we are more likely to speak up if our words are valued. This is just another of the many forms of divine communication. The Divine is whatever you wish to label it or not. The essence of all these is ultimately the same. There is no separation.

As with all life, each body is a representation of the Universe, the Earth and that which lives upon it. The body is life upon life upon life. It is your personal universe to learn from, to care for and to support. There are worms, bacteria and unseen bugs within the intestinal track. For the body-universe to feel good and to provide a quality experience, these must all be in balance. Too much sugar and the worms grow out of control; feces stick to the walls and block nutrients. The immune system gets stressed handling so much, and the individual universe becomes vulnerable to illness and disease. In the digestive chapter, I share a recipe for cleaning out stuck feces.

If the mind is not balanced in healthy thinking and properly nourished with quality energy from nutrition, the physical and energetic bodies attract charged life experiences (often harsh) to help correct the imbalance. The mind and body are not separate. However, with the mind being 90% energy, thinking is prioritized to facilitate making physical corrections. Remember that thought is energy. The brain is wired by our thinking. Neuron connections link sensory inputs and motor outputs in the various lobes of the cerebral cortex. The brain's construct is highly energetic and partly physical. Reality is formed and changed by thinking. If a person thinks negatively, the world will become negative. If others control how you think, they control the reality in which you live. Regardless of external influences, you are ultimately responsible. If changes do not happen, humanity cannot move forward. You must do the work to correct ineffective thinking.

Accepting those who live and think differently is huge to the growth of a human. There are both differences and similarities among all living creatures here on Earth and in the Universe. If you have a heart and a mind and are connected with your emotions, you are certainly human.

Diversity is in all things. Each person is dynamically different, with some similarities. For example, one body may operate at its highest performance consuming meat protein; yet another may require vegetable protein instead. It is a self-discovery process which requires people to get to know themselves on every level as much as possible, and to the highest accuracy achievable. This is a learning process which actualizes you as the person you wish to be. Keep growing because growing is healing. There are many underlying issues with societal thinking among our current and previous experiences before this life. It is complete honesty, self-integrity, compassion and love of learning. If a person wants it, they will set all motion in that direction. This is a highly individualized process.

Ever meet people so firm in their own thinking that they won't believe anything else is possible, even though you know it for a fact and can prove their position is not true? They truly and deeply believe with every fiber in their mind and body that they are right. Belief is incredibly powerful and is often dominant over a person. Have you ever broken down the meaning of words? Let's examine some word culture from the Oxford dictionary:

> **Cult**: a system of religious veneration and devotion directed toward a particular figure or object; a relatively small group of people having religious beliefs or practices regarded by others as strange or

sinister; a misplaced or excessive admiration for a particular person or thing—"a cult of personality surrounding leaders"; a person or thing that is popular or fashionable, especially among a particular section of society—"a cult film"

From the Merriam-Webster dictionary:

a religion regarded as unorthodox or spurious; great devotion to a person, idea, object, movement or work; the object of such devotion; a usually small group of people characterized by such devotion; a system of religious beliefs and ritual; formal religious veneration; a system for the cure of disease based on dogma set forth by its promulgator

Ure: forming nouns denoting an action, process or result—"censure"; forming nouns denoting an office or function—"judicature"

From the Merriam Webster dictionary:

act; process—"exposure;" office—"function;" a body performing (such) a function—"legislature"

Think about these definitions and the power held in the word "culture."

Let go of some of the unhealthy cultural, religious, organization and societal beliefs. Anything that has great influence in creating and maintaining beliefs must come into question. It does not mean each has no level of truth. It does mean that even one small piece of misinformation is all that is needed to influence and misguide. It affects your openness to learning and exploring other forms of thought, which is necessary to expand the mind and spirit! The truth about your nutrition in an ever more dominated Western world will set people free. Everything changes over time. Institutions that don't are obviously held to more than just a divine power.

Please don't shoot the messenger. It can feel deeply threatening when someone questions such institutions. Challenging these beliefs can stab the ego hard, cutting it like a knife. The ego wants to fight anything it has been trained not to accept, even when facts show otherwise. Influential institutions are mighty. Nothing escapes this until you accurately determine the truth for yourself.

Everything changes as time moves forward, and that includes truth. What is true today may very well be found to not be true tomorrow. Nothing escapes this organic reality in the earthly school. It can be challenging, but most things are when change is happening. There are a few truths that have not and likely will not change: love, compassion, acceptance of differences, kindness, ever-learning, and a divine connection for guidance and knowledge.

Did you ever sing a song you absolutely loved on the radio? You were so deeply certain of the words and the tune that you sang it over and over, only to find out years later that you had some of the words wrong. You may have felt a bit stupid or embarrassed, but you remembered the correct words from that point forward. It's just learning, but being wrong is easy. What your ears and mind heard was incorrect, yet you stuck with it until you recognized the error.

Everyone gets caught up in a belief that is not true. It's only human, and it likely happens to all life forms.

We are understanding more and more about healthy and unhealthy foods; and we are discovering new truths in the face of contradicting beliefs. Thoughts are easily altered and impressionable. There is misdirection, misinformation and intentional corruption within organizations. As a person heals, seeing this becomes much easier. The truth can be drawn out, leaving the rest behind.

Most everything in this world is designed to divide people in one form or another, even from ourselves. More often than not, excuses and triggered emotions are proffered over solutions. The Secure Profitability Formula is at play in all things, and facing this truth is of the utmost importance. Beliefs often promote a false sense of superiority by comparing beliefs, actions, race and location with others. These attitudes are supported by the false ego. They halt growth and keep people stuck. Comparison is a tragedy with no real benefit. Here's a novel idea: learn from each other! There's no pressure to be the same. It's just another viewpoint with or without value, and it adds to your journey.

Can you imagine what it might have been like if governments learned from the native tribes and incorporated their understanding, love and care for the Earth and each other?

Altering our thinking is uncomfortable. Change, evolution and growth expand our thinking and rewire the brain. It takes time, consistency, persistence and patience—and it's uncomfortable. Don't give up. Recognize the discomfort for what it is and push through. It's how our brains eventually connect the pieces.

It is impossible for every person to be skilled and knowledgeable about everything. Therefore, turning to others who have done the work and gained the knowledge and expertise can streamline and simplify the process. No single approach has all the answers. It's always a combination. Now is the time to dig deep and bring out the thoughts and experiences that hold you back. There is no more time. The world has become too toxic and too unhealthy. It needs people to step up and create the needed changes. It starts with an individual, then spreads.

This is the underlying fear of the mega-businesses because it will affect their formula. Their goals are to keep control and avoid change unless set forth by them. They will not allow freedom to step on the authoritative controls which are in place. This is simply the truth of our world. All efforts go toward influencing the generations, groups and individuals to make certain that business continues as usual. The mega-businesses are not going to let each other fail. They all have power and will ensure that none of them miss out on maintaining profits. Awareness is the first step.

Think about all the ads that show great happiness and vibrant health while shoveling *carboplunks* into their bodies. Movies enhance and encourage using harmful foods and substances. Music often evokes particular and repeatable emotions. It's designed to bring about predicted thinking followed by anticipated actions. All of this numbs the mind and is exhausting. When you negatively alter yourself, you are telling yourself you're not enough. This message is repeated in many forms, and it keeps people stuck. You are divine and you are enough.

Advertising is a powerful influencer on how people think. In these days of target advertising, it is broader and more specifically intrusive than ever before.[8] Agencies learn as much about you and your family as possible. Then they create ads whose products have a higher chance of being purchased by you. Children often want something based on an ad they saw, then pressure their parents to the extreme. There are many strategies to evoking emotions and thoughts which open up your wallet.

Here's an interesting strategy: I once sat down with a wealthy friend of mine. I asked this person to search for an item I wanted from a certain company on a popular online purchasing site. The item was identical to mine; however, this person was being charged $5 more than me. Well off or not, many people would still rather be careful with their money. We deserve not to be ripped off.

Advertising is a form of overcoming unwanted results from an unwanted reputation, regardless of the truth. One time, a doctor prescribed to me a new pain cream not yet on the market. At our next visit, he asked me his study-based questions. I answered, "It numbed the pain unless I moved; then the pain immediately came back." This product is now offered over the counter with its advertising focused on people happily moving around and having a ball, insinuating that the cream stops pain even while moving. The ingredients have not been changed. Maybe in some bodies it does

---

8 Thomas Germain, "Targeted Ads Have Come to Your TV," August 30 2021, Consumer Reports, https://www.consumerreports.org/advertising-marketing/targeted-ads-have-come-to-your-tv-a2176040919/

this, but not in mine. Claims cannot be trusted. They understand the power of thought!

A certain no-tears shampoo on the market contains a numbing ingredient, yet the product presents itself as mild. Similar products include ingredients that cause hair to fall out. Some fast-food hamburger patties are sprayed with a smoky grilled flavor to convince people it's authentically grilled. Even nice restaurants claim to be serving expensive items which are actually fake and very cheap.

The industries will continue to twist facts until they have a reason to change. Most have proven they will not. As long as we buy their products they have no reason to change anything unless it lowers profits. People believe what often gets repeated. We are giving away our freedom. It's no wonder songs repeat the same lines over and over, or that they encode subliminal messages. It works. This is a sad and undeniable truth.

Think outside the box. I was once in a grocery store with my bestie girlfriend. They were offering a big bowl of tasty guacamole and chips. I took one chip, piled a good tablespoon or two of guacamole on it and ate it. It was wonderful. I was hungry and knew the guacamole would help ease the pangs in a healthy way. By the way, being hungry in a grocery store can lead to impulsive and crappy purchases. My girlfriend considered what I did to be greedy and rather distasteful. I did not respond, but stood there watching. By the time she had a fourth chip with a socially acceptable amount of dip on each, I spoke up. "I had one chip and the same amount of dip as you. It was very satisfying, and I did not plop four fatty and salty chips into my body—only one."

Ever since, she has done the same. Who says you must have a bunch of chips to enjoy a dip, anyway? Why not have just one, pile on the dip, and walk away satisfied? Of course, this depends on the circumstances. The store had plenty of guacamole, so it wasn't like there was barely enough to go around. Live in wisdom and be respectful.

One day, I watched as my daughter-in-law handed half an avocado and a spoon to my grandson (nature is simple). He gobbled it down without adding a thing. It was gorgeous to watch. No doubt others do this, but I had never seen it before. We learn from each other, and especially from those who think outside the societally designed cage. It opens our minds to new ideas that can serve us better. We help each other and we need each other. We need you, too!

Not everyone is meant to heal. In my world, most everyone chooses to learn specific lessons on this Earth. If part of that lesson is to experience a health issue, then so be it. Even so, nutrition can lessen the impact. It can also reduce possible feelings of guilt as you aid the body.

Be realistic. A *carboplunk* for a tasty treat once in a while is amazing. Enjoy it to the max. Then get back to your goal and on track. Repeating this later that day or the next day only leads to more undermining indulgences before addiction starts to take over. How many times have you lost a bit of weight, only to reach for these items and gain it back? They are meant to be addictive. Embrace this new you and don't argue with it. The decision is for nutrition with flexibility and adaptability.

When you go to a dinner party and refuse to eat anything, claiming you are only eating healthy, it can come across as rude and disrespectful. Talking about it is unnecessary. Instead, take a healthy dish to share (unless you're indulging). I have often observed a brilliant friend of mine taking a nice big salad to a gathering and being the only one to eat it. She inspires me to do the same. I found this to be a source of strength. It can be a most satisfying experience. This is not a comparison to others, but a decision to aid the body in nutrition and spirit in fun and healthy ways. Choose your poisons carefully.

These concepts are intended to help you make better choices, to be more in tune as a listener, and to be an avid supporter of the body. Stop being such a harsh self-judger. Instead, get lovingly reconnected with what this body can do for us. None of this is possible unless you have the desire to change.

Forgiveness.

Buried emotions must be discovered. Resentment, grief, trauma, shame, guilt, fear, embarrassment, humiliation, blame and similar emotions derived from experiences all require forgiveness—not for the other person, but for you. You don't need to forget them, but you can let go of your attachments with compassion, understanding, kindness and love. Thoughts that involve harming the self or someone harming you can be hard to get past. Understanding can be a challenge. Holding onto the judgment and blame is damaging to you.

There is an energetic and physical response to the trauma you suffer. For example, insurance claims and legal actions can drag on and on, requesting the same information over and over. This is designed to have the victim experience trauma over and over. They do it because it works, and it has devastating effects. Every time you think of the experience, it's as if you are reliving it all over again. It's a Post Traumatic Stress Disorder (PTSD).[9]

It can be a very hard pill to swallow when your choices put you in a situation that is life-threatening, harsh, and where escape seems overwhelming. Your choice could also be self-damaging, as with an addiction. It is painful. Sometimes you can bury this type of pain so deep that you have no idea why you react the way you do.

As mentioned earlier, seek help to get this resolved so you can find ways to forgive and let go. Your thinking may not have had any effect on attracting such experiences. People can get caught up in someone else's karma, and accidents happen.

When I was nine years old, I had three serious infections: lung, bladder and kidney. I won't go into the story at this time, but I died. While on the other side, I learned that my mother and participating father were not expected to become so abusive. Unexpected results happen in a life plan. Those on the other side of this life are also learning about creation. They do not have all the answers. This is how I know for a fact that accidents happen, that people can get harmed through no fault of their own.

Lighten up on yourself, get help and find ways to heal. Listen to Dr. Joe Dispenza's *Forgiveness* videos on YouTube.

---

9 Matthew Tull, PhD and medically reviewed by Daniel B. Block, MD, "Types of Re-Experiences in PTSD," November 16, 202, verywell mind, https://www.verywellmind.com/re-experiencing-2797325

His presentations are outstanding, and he knows this subject well. You may also wish to check out what Leland Holgate is doing. He is no longer a quadriplegic. Don't give up. Keep seeking professional and higher quality (most religious counselors and leaders are NOT qualified) assistance until you can get on healthier ground. If I can do it with the many extremes in my life, so can you.

Powerful desire.

Desire is not an emotion, but it's similar to feelings. Combining thought and experience creates desire, which is a physical and neurological reaction. It is a specific state of mind.[10] For example, when an unhealthy addiction takes over, there is recognition with the experience that connects a thought. It causes chemicals to react in the brain, which affects the nerves so that an emotional/physical desire occurs. Each time a person chooses to satisfy this craving, it reinforces the experience with thoughts. Desire and cravings then set in. Thought must change first so the feeling of desire is more in line with your goals. Desire, passion and hunger have strong influences in attracting more learning experiences into life. Emotion is incredibly strong. They are also a form of communication about thinking.

In early childhood, people often learn to shut off feelings. They are told not to show them or trust them, or that somehow feelings mean nothing. In truth, feelings and emotions are required for influencing or manifesting. They are a form of divine communication. Feelings are highly attached to

---

10 Stanford Encyclopedia of Philosophy, "Desire," December 9 2009, revised April 9 2015, https://plato.stanford.edu/entries/desire/

beliefs, both working and not working. How many wealthy people have you heard say that money is evil? Many poor people believe this. Some believe genetics determine all the power and that individuals are at their mercy. None of these beliefs are true. Both have influence, and both are just excuses to avoid taking responsibility and make necessary changes.

Want to make the world change? Each individual must *be* the change. Ignite the brain so it starts rewiring itself right now. Each body vibrates, and vibrating healthy choice attracts the same. A person may feel something, but it does not mean it is a truthful feeling. Some powerful feelings, like love, require logic. Always involve the brain and the heart. The heart has its own intelligence, and it's our connection to the divine and all that is. It can analyze vibration in a way the brain cannot. Both need to be used. Both are required for understanding and creating healthier desires.

Eastern philosophy has always regarded our organs as having their own intelligence. *Hug and take care of your heart. It is gentle and precious. Don't damage it with negativity.* In hypnotherapy, a quality practitioner can literally have you talk directly with your heart, or anything else within the body, to ascertain what it needs to heal and be at optimum health. Don't avoid getting a physical and blood test from time to time. These can clue you into needed life changes.

Thank your heart for being so sweet and kind. It thinks, acts, reacts and remembers what you feed it emotionally and physically. Let it know you are making changes, and let it guide you with love and kindness. It is in a relationship with you.

Kitchen and home cleanliness.

There are medical and scientific reasons for keeping a home and kitchen area clean. Bacteria and germs form in dirty places and float through the air. The immune system can get overloaded, weakening it and causing illness. A clean-as-you-go concept can be most helpful. By the time a meal is ready, most of the cleanup would be done, leaving only table dishes, food storage and serving dishes.

Condiments and dairy products should be put away immediately after using and before sitting down to eat. They last much longer and stay fresher this way. Never leave them out. Every part of the clean-as-you-go process will make it easier to finish.

There are times when things get behind. Working, volunteering, shopping, cooking, cleaning, school, appointments, yard work, sports, bills to pay, other chores and the like can become overwhelming. It's going to happen. Keep these things in mind and clean in small amounts. Keep at it until things get caught up. Health is worth it. Hopefully, as children get older these become easier. Children should observe adults being helpful, appreciative and forgiving so they can also value the efforts of making meals and such. Always find opportunities to say thank you and please.

Keep the home organized and do consistent cleaning. Knowing where to find things is less stressful, and this aids health. It also improves organizing other areas of life. Finish tasks as often as you can. Leaving things partially done adds up quickly and only increases chaotic energies. Vibrations attract like vibrations. Be grateful and respectful for a place to live.

And clean out the clutter! Too much unused stuff is simply a waste, and it gets in the way. It creates stuck and stagnant frequencies.

Awareness.

Maintain a mindful awareness. Get out of your head, do what needs to be done, face the truth, takes steps to solve, be aware of passing thoughts and sensations, and stay in the moment at hand. All this can provide helpful information. Focus on short-term and long-term tasks until you've completed as much as possible. When the mind wanders, focus is lost. You are no longer present with what is being done, and the opportunity to learn and help others can slip by. Being present is an art in itself. It can help bring in unexpected solutions, deeper awareness, and supports appreciation and gratefulness. Do everything with excellence. Skip the perfection ideal. Just do your best at most everything you do. This is respectfulness and appreciation for experience and learning.

Whether we recognize it or not, every action and reaction has an emotion attached to it. When these emotions are not acknowledged, they can appear in other areas, causing you to wonder what happened. Get some help to better recognize and increase the tools needed for further healing and development. Review the archetypes at the back of this book to help expand your knowledge and give you words to better define feelings, emotions and parts of your personality.

A qualified therapist can aid in providing a process to recognize emotions and give them their space, letting go of those that do not serve us. The process can be customized to a person; but overall, it delivers meaningful insights and experiences. Many emotions can get complicated. We tend to deny or accept those that demand more of our attention. Emotions are of the Divine. They are incredible in communicating what works and what does not. As we work with them, we become closer to the spiritual beings we truly are. This is where our real power lies.

Taking quality care of yourself is beautiful, exciting, healing and joyful. It's a healthy way to thrive in a chaotic, confusing and downright weird world. Let's take a big step forward and reboot, reclaim and revise our nutritional thinking. Let's eradicate denial and make this an adventure in self-discovery. Put your personal power where it really belongs: in your hands!

Teach your body to support the new thinking.

We chose to teach our body when and what to crave: eat when happy, eat when bored, eat when sad. When we ignore certain emotions, we create feelings of being deprived, thinking that life is unfair or that others have it easier. Stop comparing yourself to others. It's just an excuse to avoid working on you.

Speak with the body. It has intelligence. Let it know you are making changes and keep reminding it of these changes. Talk with it. Have patience as it adjusts to the new you. Adjustment could take years, so it's unfair to expect it to immediately realize what you are doing. It's your baby, so be gentle and communicate kindly. Do away with expectations and get present with what can be learned. Thank the body for its support and for making these changes with you. It will surprise you how affective this technique is. Nothing likes to be taken for granted, including the body. It has survived what you have put it through thus far, and it deserves respect.

Oh, the rewards.

Expecting a reward is unrealistic. If a person expects to be rewarded with 10 pounds of weight lost every week, they are likely to fail. The inveterate reward is the new relationship with the body and how it will respond and support you—whether or not you lose weight.

The body tends to accept and become comfortable with a particular weight range. If you were comfortable in that range for a while, the body regulated you there. This is called a set point. The body needs time to reckon when you may be wandering away from this once happy place. You may lose weight quickly at some point, but not at all at other times. Congratulatory pats on the back are great, but keep them in alignment. Enjoy them but don't expect them.

Healing steps.

There must be healing before lasting change. Those who have healed their physical bodies have consistently done these things:

- Drastically changed their diet
- Took control of personal health by letting go of excuses
- Used intuition
- Used herbs and supplements
- Released deep-seated emotions
- Raised positive emotions
- Incorporated social support
- Increased and deepened spiritual connection
- Had a strong reason for living

When you practice all these things, you get rid of what is not working and get in tune with what is working. You pay attention to what is happening *right now*. The past is in the past. The future is not yet here, but we're working toward it. We are living in the moment.

STOP IT!

Stop living life through the television. Stop living life through technology. Create and live your own story. Get out in nature. Build a life you are excited about. When the technology babysitters are no longer needed, they will have less impact on you. Stop merely surviving and *live*. Stop watching others live a fake and scripted life through a television screen. Stop watching from the sidelines. Become a story that can be lived, not just watched.

Intuition/psychic.

All religions and belief systems speak of their role models having the skill to get messages from beyond for guidance, healing and warnings. Regain this skill and use it. Seek out those who believe you have the same abilities. You are divine and have within you the bright, white spark of Source. You may see this when very relaxed. It could be as small as the tip of a needle, but it is there. I do this for my clients and also to aid the unseen in safely moving on to the other side. One of the easiest ways to tell when you may be getting an intuitive message is when it's out of context with what a person is thinking, doing or saying at the time. It could be something like, *Huh? That's interesting.*

Think back to a time when the hair on the back of your neck stood up, warning you about something life-threatening, or when you felt a tightness and heaviness in the pit of your stomach. Those were intuitive communications. They are stronger in some people, depending on the eternal advancements within each.

Many of our young people are coming into this world with highly developed psychic skills. Those wishing to develop these skills must learn the Universal rules that apply to using this natural ability. Understanding the different forms, how to use them and how to analyze them (as in dreams and visions) are highly important. Seek out qualified and experienced individuals. There are many like me who offer coaching classes and books on the subject. Some people may only have one skill, such as clairvoyance (seeing in the mind or having visions); others may have all the skills. For example, my clairsentience (feeling shifts in energy and having the ability to define them accurately) is the most developed of all my skills.

Keep in mind we each have our own view of the world based on our life experiences. There may be similar views, but they aren't necessarily the same ones. Views can play a role in how to interpret and share this information. There are common mistakes psychics can make because of this. For example, I may see you moving *to* California, while others see you *in* California. The ability to accurately discern information is a valuable skill in a highly tuned intuitive.

Visualizing gift technique.

Visualization can make life changes easy, fun and highly effective. Hug your precious and loving heart throughout the day. Flood your energy and physical body with love, compassion and kindness. Create an imaginary box filled with gifts such as chocolates, flowers, certificates, money—anything another person would like. These energetic gifts can actually help to satisfy the energy of another. Ultimately, these imaginary gifts are a piece of energetic love.

One day, I was pulled over by a policeman after being caught speeding. A ticket was the last thing I needed. He was very cocky in his actions. Rather than slip into anger mode or figure out how I could avoid a ticket, I chose to envision energetic gifts. This is something I learned decades ago to ease energy with someone and/or a situation. Speaking with the officer, it put my mind in a place where it didn't react to the ticket or the situation. It gave me the opportunity to influence the energy with a form of love. In a healthy mindset, giving a gift (energetically or physically) is based in love. Eventually, the officer gave me a ticket because his supervisor told him to write one. They were concerned about the number of accidents that had been occurring in that area. When I looked at the ticket, I noticed he wrote it for 5 mph over the limit. I had been going 15 over! His initial actions as he approached my car made it clear he was the authority. In the end, he helped me out. I have seen this visualization technique work many times. Even though it did not alter my results, it changed my thinking and helped me handle the situation without defensive or fearful emotions.

Place gifts in doorways, homes, offices and cars. This is a great way to alter negative attitudes. The energy of the other person becomes calmer and more satisfied. Feel the empty space and fill it up. Then turn it over to your celestial team (your guide, guardians and angels who aid you in this life).

We do not use them enough, and they are here to help. They are the small nudge or voice that gives guidance. I sometimes argue with them, but most often they are absolutely right. It is human to question, after all.

Emotional communication.

Emotion is another form of divine communication. Let's say Mike realizes that he gets easily irritated by others. This interferes with relationships and quells a desire to change. To change, he must notice exactly what triggers the recurring anger and frustration. As he observes, Mike notices that whenever a person expresses a contrary opinion he gets frustrated and angry. He blames the other person because they were the cause of his frustration which led to anger. Mike has learned that no one can make him feel anything. He now tries to define the emotion that rises up just before anger. The emotion he feels comes from being offended. Why should he care about what others choose to think?

Mike now sits with this feeling, gives it space, clears all thought and just allows the emotion to speak. He realizes he is afraid of being wrong and is threatened by another's opinion. This is based in the ego wanting to feel superior, comparing what he believes to the other and the need to be right over all else. Each time this situation arises, Mike is observing what emotion comes up and what thinking is attached to it. The next time he notices his insecurity—another valuable emotion. He realizes he repeated another's opinion and did not research it for accuracy. Mike then does the research and tweaks his opinion to be more accurate.

He now feels firm in stating his opinion. But wait! Another

emotion arises. This time it's the need to feel right. He discovers that the other person's point is reasonable. He had not asked why the person saw the subject in that way. How can a person grow and expand if they do not ask questions?

The next time this subject comes up, he makes a point to ask why. When the other person explains why and how she came to her opinion, it is fully evident her view also has truth. Every single person has a different view of things. No one stands in the same place with the same experiences and the same information to form an opinion. Asking questions leads to uncovering a whole different way to look at any given subject. It may support your own stance, part of it, or be totally different.

When the process was completed, many thoughts were changed and realigned with the new thinking of not having to be right. Mike was missing out on valuable learning and expanding his own knowledge. Surprisingly, he had been thinking the same thing about the other person. Often, when one person feels a certain way, the other is likely feeling the same. Each thought the other was closed-minded and a know-it-all. This led to both not listening, not asking questions and being stuck in the mud with their thinking.

This process reveals what we never expected about ourselves. It continues until thinking eventually becomes aligned. An emotion clues us into thinking, which leads us to acting and reacting in a way that does not work. Then another emotion rises and does the same. Positive actions and reactions are much more supportive to a person who is open to hearing other views, considering and altering their own views as needed. This process repeats for everything.

It cascades throughout until the thinking occurs from every angle. This process is another form of divine communication. Emotions clue us into the thinking that works and the thinking that holds us back.

It is during this process that many give up, but please don't! It gets easier and easier. Practice and experience are necessary. It is a natural self-evolution. Eventually, the troubled thinking is changed at all levels. Natural expansion takes over and introduces new trains of thought which must go through this very process. We become closer and closer to our own truth and stay open to change, more easily recognizing the guidance that makes our lives much easier.

Change is fearful. It can be debilitating. Changing our thinking is always uncomfortable. The brain expands, reigniting parts that were not being used. Embracing this process of change is highly liberating and can be exciting. Think of it as a type of self-improvement detective game.

We are all connected, and we need each other. Getting real with the self, changing ways of thinking and how we act and react can teach others better than words ever can. We are here to learn this as part of our positive progression. A benefit to this is that a person becomes more focused on learning and realignment. Moving forward is much easier. In the example above, the other person felt accepted and valued instead of defensive and threatened. Mike then had a new understanding and a new friend.

2| Getting Real

Dump excuses.

There are no excuses like age or genetics. Eating healthily is not hard. There is great joy in knowing you are taking good care of something that is so personally supportive and valuable. Age, genetics and time have an effect, but very little if the thinking and actions are in line. Going through a fast-food line takes more time than tossing an apple to the kid in the back seat. I get it that life can be overwhelming and busy. Sometimes we just want a break or want someone else to help us for a change. Get the kids involved in cooking. This is where technology can be most helpful and constructive. We should all have some cooking and meal preparation skills. Simplifying is natural, and it doesn't require a ton of spices or added flavorings. Salt and sugar are used so abundantly that people can find natural nutrition less appealing. Face what must be faced and correct whatever thought is behind it. This is true freedom. Heal first, get healthier at every level, and the rest will follow.

A kind and loving friend of mine deeply believed that when there was a break at her work, she absolutely had to go to the snack machines to get a *carboplunk*. With two breaks and a lunch period every day, those *carboplunks* add up quickly.

An obese relative shared with me that she was not obligated by anyone to do anything as long as she was eating. No one expected her to work, and this gave her an excuse to not feel guilty about it. Her rule of thumb is to eat three meals a day plus snacks. In private, she battled depression, never facing the emotions that troubled her. I observed other relatives buy cases and cases of diet soda. Buying into the fantasy of a quick and easy weight fix, they tried every fad diet that came around. They ate when bored, happy or sad. We create desires that support our actions. Addiction comes in many forms—excuses being one of them.

I have heard many comments from clients. *I have no time. It's easier to grab fast food than make my hungry kids wait until we get home. Cooking messes up the kitchen and takes too much planning. If it doesn't come out of a can or box, I won't do it.* I get it. Preparing and clean-up are not enjoyable chores; but if you wish to eat well and consume healthy foods, it's necessary.

With every generation, children struggle more and more with adult diseases and weight issues. Children raised on foods and beverages with little nutrients and lots of salt and sugars will struggle with their health as adults. What they grew up with makes it even harder to create change. In past Native American culture, many adults did not feed their children anything too tasty, opting for bland foods until they're around 8 years old. This made it much easier for them as adults to fall back on the bland diet to aid the body in healing when sick. A bland diet allows the body to use precious energy toward healing rather than digesting. This action is responsible and loving. This what parenting is all about. Helping the child build a foundation makes it easier to face life struggles and thrive.

Instead of going to a fast-food place, try grabbing from a bag of apples before picking up the kids. Handing them an apple takes far less time and is inexpensive. Eating from the earth is easy. Making a salad does not require a dozen items. Two scrambled eggs are easier and less messy than making bacon, pancakes or sausage. It can be very simple. It does, however, require a bit more planning. Parents have the most responsibility for food choices. It takes the leaders of the home to not only make a healthy team but *be* the role model.

It takes a team! Everyone should be participating in the eats. No person is subordinate in this area. If both parents work, they should both participate. Either can easily cook on a weekend, help with cleanup, put together a simple salad or chop a single onion. All household members can be supporting and participating in whatever is needed.

Get the kids involved; they need not be catered to. For ideas, find creative counseling, talk to a skilled and respected teacher, or even find a support group. Use psychology! Get them involved so everyone benefits.

I love the story of a wise woman who filled her plate with vegetables and gave her young children only the protein. It did not take long for them to ask why her plate was different. She stated that the vegetables were adult food, then she hesitantly let them try some. They grew up loving vegetables. Growing vegetables can be simple and fun for children. A pot of lettuce in a home is easy to grow, or maybe an herb like rosemary. It has been scientifically proven that plants have thoughts and feelings. They react and thrive with love, and shrivel in an environment with hate and anger. Teaching love for other life, especially life that supports survival, is great awareness for parents and caretakers.

Get creative. Read and do the work to solve a problem. When something works, share it with others. Teaching kids to cook is not hard; the cleanup is another matter. The best advice I can give is to clean as you go. Kids get overwhelmed just like adults. If there's less mess, there will likely be greater acceptance for the cleanup. Meal time is such a wonderful part of connecting to people here and around the world. Looking up recipes online and learning how to prepare many things is a gift which can be used to streamline healthier, successful and unique approaches. Learn about it and participate!

Eat your words.

Words have their own measurable vibrations. We place additional energetic vibrations on words through our intentions. You've probably heard this: *Don't say I'll try; instead, say I'm doing!* The word *try* means you may or may not; it gives an option. When the words *am doing* are used, there is no option. Make your decisions and don't argue with them. Repeat to yourself that the decision is final! Many studies have proven the success of these, over and over. Let's use them to our advantage.

To break an unhealthy eating habit like fast food, I have found the word *poison* to be highly affective. In the past, every time I drove past a fast-food location that tempted me, I would say *poison* to myself. Over time, it helped break such cravings. The use of this word has great power. It touches the deepest and most basic survival aspect of ourselves. Everyone recognizes the power of this word. This is not a new concept. I have used it in this manner ever since.

Stop using negative words. All of us are guilty of this. How many times have we called ourselves stupid, an idiot or something similar! We are the source of all creation. We are divine energy and spirit living a physical existence. There is much credence in using appropriate words for a life of thriving and love. People thrive in a loving environment and shrivel in an environment of hate. Refuse to separate and divide yourself from the Divine.

The written word has greater power than the spoken word. At the end of every day, write down what you are grateful for. List the little things that can get muddled up in the confusion and frustrations of the world. Keep it simple. Written words having a long-lasting vibration. In the space of gratefulness, much positivity can happen. Some would even say that magic happens.

Words repeatedly spoken drive themselves into your soul. The written word has an even stronger vibration. This can be used to help shift away from self-destructive thinking. This is why affirmations are so effective. Repeating words for emotional and spiritual support can help us focus and create desired change. Here are some phrases I often use in hypnotherapy sessions:

- I believe in me.
- Every bite of nutritious food feeds my body and soul.
- I am focusing my emotions to train my body and empower energy.
- I am my dream.
- Exercise is fun, and my body reacts by becoming stronger.
- All I think and do is supportive of love.
- My heart is precious; it is a gift.
- The words I think and say are loving, kind and supportive of health.
- Every change I am making is in support of my healthier self.
- I am kind and compassionate with myself and others.
- I am perfectly imperfect; it is good.
- Everything I put in my mouth is in support of all that is me.
- I choose what I put in my mouth.
- I embrace making my own decisions.
- I can and I am.
- My actions support my goals.
- Doing is joy.
- I love choosing healthy nutrition.
- I speak and think supporting and loving words.
- I set my intent every day with these affirmations.
- This awareness leads to healing and is just a step toward joyful *be-ing*.
- I believe in me.

You want to what? Really?

It can be difficult if some in the household insist on fast food and *carboplunks*. It's counterproductive when a partner offers you unhealthy food in hopes of having someone to share it with. Not all partners are capable of supporting another's choice. There must be freedom in relationships. It's wonderful when a couple can work together.

Some partners have more controlling and undermining motives. These types of personalities are more challenging. I know of someone who wanted the other partner to gain weight so that person would no longer be considered attractive to others. Some partners may simply want the sheer pleasure of knowing they are influencing and causing a desired reaction. Then there are those who take pleasure in their partners' failures in order to boost their own insecurities.

Our own actions determine the outcome. We cannot change an unwilling person who shares our surroundings, but we can rise above these tactics while respecting their beliefs. A quality professional can be a great source of alternative thinking. The goal is that you do not harm yourself and that you learn tactics which help you safely reach your goals.

I have a treasured friend who values her health. For many years, I witnessed her serve questionable meals to her partner and healthy ones to herself. After getting guidance from a therapist, she no longer reacted emotionally to this. She would serve herself a salad with protein while serving her partner's protein on a bun with heavy condiments, chips and a sugary side. Another friend simply served what she wanted for herself while her partner altered whatever he wished. She was determined not to cater to someone else. Her partner was able to remove, add, or just make for himself whatever he liked.

If we really want something, we will find a way to do it. Partners can and do get on the same page. Getting external guidance can really help. Consistently accommodating a partner, especially at the beginning of a relationship, is very hard to maintain. Keep this in mind. It's not fair to start a relationship by doing so much, then later decide to change things. Each should find ways to help make it easier on the other.

Seriously.

Everyone needs nutrition every day, right? Self-sufficiency is most helpful. Depending on others to purchase and prepare allows them to choose and handle what gets put in your mouth. Salad dressings are simple and inexpensive to make: cider vinegar, Himalayan pink sea salt, honey, olive oil and mustard—all the savory sweet, sour, salty and fat in proper portions. It's amazing dressing. Fresh lemon juice with garlic is an outstanding marinade for chicken. There are many online resources and books for simple recipes. The body needs variety, so don't get stuck doing the same meals week after week. Change it up a bit. A baby food grinder is a cheap way to share healthfully prepared foods for those needing ground foods. It's not easy, but do what you can.

When my children were around 7 and 8 years old, I remember being at a grocery store one day. They were charged with looking for something new in the fruit and vegetable department. It was a very interesting time and lasted only a few months, but it allowed them to try new things. They had a lot of fun doing this and it was a pleasure to watch. Children love participating in the eats if given the opportunity. They also get to see their parents trying something new.

Teaching children to follow a recipe is not difficult. As the recipes get more involved it can be a challenge. For a year, my children had the opportunity to choose one meal to make every other week. They would choose a recipe and make a grocery list, then we'd head off to the store. They learned to read labels, use coupons, test for freshness, and so on. These were the basics of meal preparation, storage and purchasing.

When the oldest entered 9th grade and the youngest was in 7th, I required them to make their own lunches. I gave each of them cash in the equivalent amount of their school lunch money. After three weeks, they were going through ads together and cutting out coupons. Their combined efforts cut costs, and they had a few extra dollars to pocket. I was very proud of them because they learned many lessons. I watched them struggle with decisions and figure out how to solve any problems that came up.

Get involved in organizations, talk to teachers, research online, find videos, get children's cookbooks, etc. Be creative and find ways to help kids learn this valuable skill.

But… it's social.

Celebrations can be just another excuse to eat *carboplunks*; but there's no need to feel pressured to eat sugary cake, doughnuts or the like. It doesn't matter what others choose, and there are usually better options. A burger patty can be eaten without the bun. Skip the potato salad and bring a healthy salad or vegetable.

Once, at an office party, alcohol was flowing like water. I watched as coworkers got smashed. They made certain I always had a drink in my hand. I accepted, but many got thrown down the sink when no one was looking. After that experience, I researched alcoholic-looking beverages. I like lemon-lime sodas on rare occasions. A lime slice also floats nicely in the glass. It's tasty and refreshing, and I can sip it over a long period of time. Ginger beer is another option that does not contain alcohol. This beverage is carbonated and has a sprig of mint. I will share later another amazing non-alcoholic, energizing and detoxifying drink.

When attending a dinner party, bring a healthy dish to share. Once, at an all-day conference, I chose to go to the nearby healthy grocery store for lunch. I purchased a piece of fruit, an avocado and two single-serving cheeses while most everyone else went to fast-food places. Avoiding the fast-food coma by eating a salad or other healthy choices is highly satisfying. You will feel alert, energized and focused for the rest of the afternoon. It's fun and incredibly satisfying to find ways to support the body in a healthy lifestyle.

The point here is to never be rude to people; but at the same time, don't allow others to control what you put in your mouth. There are many other choices. There's absolutely no reason you can't find easy and tasty solutions.

Do you see it?

Visualization can be highly effective when done honestly and correctly. Be loving toward yourself: Hug that amazing and loving heart throughout the day, because it is so very precious. Practice flooding your energy and physical body with love, compassion and kindness. See yourself active, vibrant, feeling strong and healthy. In your mind, see yourself enjoying nutritious items. See them traveling throughout your powerful body as it gets what it needs for its highest functioning level. Feel it, hug it and communicate with it. Be appreciative and have trust in its ability to adapt.

Your body is meant to serve you. See it getting healthier and healthier. Observe it moving freely as you play in a park and go for a walk. See how the skin glows, the hair shines and the nails grow. Make it realistic!

In your mind, put a mirror in front of your body. See yourself looking back at you. Now, tell your body how amazing it is and thank it for serving you so well. Tell it you are making changes to support you. See it morph into a healthier body. Imagine tiny miners throughout your body as their tools chip away unnecessary cholesterol. Visualization is how a person communicates with the subconscious mind. It aligns the mind, body and spirit. It's also a form of meditation because it sets intention and informs the body. Loving it elicits response and cooperation.

Design a vision board. Determine your ideal health by using lovely pictures of healthy items. Draw pictures of being connected with your body. Diffuse the negativity that says we are not good enough. Use images that would support your efforts. How about a day at the hot springs, or maybe a massage? What about flowers? Keep it simple.

Heart and mind matter.

Media impacts the mind, which affects how the heart perceives. The heart can be in error when your mind is in error. If the thinking is negative, the heart responds and will have negative input and output. They work together. This is another reason to correct thinking. Many have difficulty seeing beyond their own experience, and this can lead to a lack of empathy. With healthy thinking (mind and heart working together) and increased empathy (sensing and understanding the feelings of others), the immune system strengthens. Bigotry, malice and sense of privilege weaken the immune system, making it more vulnerable to illness and disease. When healthy, the system operates at the same rhythm and vibration.[11]

The subconscious mind remembers everything. It never stops taking in information and stores every single bit it receives. Every experience, here and beyond this life, is stored within. It is a supercomputer. It does not differentiate between truth and fiction, but your conscious mind will. Have you ever experienced something and just *knew* it wasn't right? That's the subconscious mind pointing out a flaw in the conscious mind's interpretation.

The subconscious mind can process 207,000,000 bits of information per second. The conscious mind only processes 40 bits of information per second (*The Biology of Belief*, Lipton, 2000). These figures may differ depending on the researcher. In my opinion, the word *process* is used very

---

11 Johan Cools, "Counter-Hacking the Subconscious Mind: Antidote for Faulty Human Perceptions From the Media Sphere," 2022, IGI Global Publisher of Timely Knowledge, https://www.igi-global.com/chapter/counter-hacking-the-subconscious-mind/296559

loosely. The subconscious holds all the information but does not necessarily interpret it. The conscious mind is needed to help connect the pieces. The conscious mind is the observer and can also discern right from wrong. It has an inferior processing capacity than the subconscious mind.[12] However, both must work together for efficient processing. The subconscious can tell if the stored information makes sense or not, but with so much information in there to process it can often be inaccurate. This is why so much effort is placed on repetitive and subliminal (visual and audible) messages. If the subconscious mind can be influenced, then underlying thinking and behavior can be influenced whether the conscious mind recognizes it or not. Ever buy something impulsively, only to regret it and wonder why you did? There are many layers to consider, accurately or inaccurately.

When the subconscious combines experiences, emotions and conscious thinking affected by trauma, it can get overwhelmed with information and trigger conditions such as Post Traumatic Stress Disorder (PTSD), which is a normal reaction to an abnormal situation. It's the brain trying to protect you. It can connect and conclude in ways that are disruptive to your behavior and life. Watching, learning and being able to recognize things all depend on your subconscious state of mind.[13]

Emotion sends signals to the brain. Every cell adjusts

---

12 Johan Cools, "Counter-Hacking the Subconscious Mind: Antidote for Faulty Human Perceptions From the Media Sphere," 2022, IGI Global Publisher of Timely Knowledge, https://www.igi-global.com/chapter/counter-hacking-the-subconscious-mind/296559

13 Savita P Patil, Deep shikha Jakhwal, Shipra Gupta, Kumud Pant, 2021. "Intersecting behavior through patterns of subconscious,". Journal of Medicine, P'ceutical & Allied. Sci. V 10 - S 2, 2034, P- 117-119. doi: 10.22270/jmpas.2021.V10S2.2034.

to the released chemicals. The nervous system then tells the body how to react to the thinking behind the emotion and the world around us. Emotion is a powerful communicator that can clue you into thinking what may not be supportive. When trauma occurs, the emotional process causes the body to relive the experience.

The conscious mind needs access to the many pieces of information stored in the subconscious mind. It sifts through and extracts what's best for healing the skewed thinking and omits the rest. There are many rooms and floors in the mansions of the mind.

In hypnotherapy, the subconscious is accessed for information so that the mind, body and spirit can be recalibrated and aligned. It is a successful way of utilizing the energy/spirit mind to consciously correct the willing (yet confused) subconscious mind.

When dreaming, the subconscious mind uses imagery which is aided by the guidance of the spirit mind. This enables the conscious mind to collate the pieces, which can help discern their meaning. There are many kinds of dreams, including release dreams which let go of unwanted and frustrating emotions and dreams that warn of selfishness. Dream study is fascinating and worth checking into. Dreaming is healthy. It's full of guidance and information intended to reestablish balance. Western science has yet to recognize the energy/spirit mind formally and openly.

Sleep.

Sleep is very broad and highly important to health and well-being. Sleep has many disruptions such as frequencies and vibrations in the air, electrical equipment, toxins, lack of proper nutrition, food sensitivities and exercise. Two of the biggest disrupters are hidden emotion and the denial of an emotion connected to a traumatic or negatively influencing experience. It is buried so deeply that there is no conscious awareness of it. When a person with this issue tries to relax, stress rises in the body from this unresolved issue.

Studies show that light affects sleep. Try to use full spectrum lighting in areas where you spend most of your time. The unseen color aids in balancing hormones. When tested in classrooms, teachers went home energized instead of drained, and the students' grades went up two levels. Full spectrum lighting affects mood, ability to function, shows objects as they appear, reduces eye fatigue, and has psychological and physiological benefits.[14]

When speaking with Mr. Seth Davis, a certified adult sleep coach and owner of Sleepably in Denver, Colorado, he stated that sleep is very connected to the balance in your lives. Once sleep is troubled, the mind can get stuck thinking that sleep will not happen. He believes 80-85% of this is in the mind. Worry, stress and how you think about sleep are very impactful. It can also become a lower priority. Sleepably looks at the balance in all levels of your life to aid in pinpointing what is out of balance in energy, life, thoughts and nutrition.

Genetics can affect sleep, but it does not shape your iden-

---

14 April Baumgartner Snethen, "EFFECTS OF FULL-SPECTRUM LIGHTING ON USE OF CLASSROOM LIBRARY CENTER BY PRESCHOOL CHILDREN," 1995, chrome-extension://efaidnbmnnnibpcajpcglclefindmkaj/https://vitamindwiki.com/tiki-download_wiki_attachment.php?attId=1882

tity. Get past these beliefs. Seth also agrees that less light in the bedroom is better. Taking a sleep aid is a crutch, and it's not a healthy choice. They are meant for short-term use and have side effects, and you can quickly build up a tolerance. There are no magic pills or medicines that solve this issue.

Explore possibilities and techniques that can put you in the correct mindset to improve behaviors around sleep. Lack of sleep is frustrating and puts people in an unhealthy mental state. We need and learn from each other. It all is part of our path of healing and growth. Check out the quality businesses focused on aiding people in overcoming what is not working. Also, it's never wise to go to bed with a full stomach. It disrupts sleep; the body does its most impactive healing while you sleep.

Get nosy, exercise and hydrate.

When I smell yummy things, I let my nose taste it. I know my body does not need to have anything at that time. Smell is amazing and it has no calories. Breathe it in, fill the lungs and send it out into the bloodstream. We taste more with our noses than our tongues. Do something physical like going for a walk, exercising or busying the hands. Drink something hydrating. We often allow others to make choices for us. You have freedom of choice, so make it fun and choose wisely. If not you, then who?

Purified clean water is the most important fluid. It flushes and cleanses the body. When you first wake up and before drinking any other beverage, drink 8-10 ounces of water. This will flush toxins and buildup from the all-important kidneys. Lessen things that dry out the body such as tea, coffee and alcohol. Sugary, fake-colored beverages are not treats and do not properly hydrate. Water is the first and foremost choice for your amazing body. Be sure to eat your vegetables so you get the necessary minerals from the earth for hydration absorption. Purifying water removes many, if not all, of these.

This is something my parents did well for their children. We drank water at nearly every meal. I hated milk and was rightfully appalled at their carbonated diet beverages, so these were never tempting to me. My children and grandchildren were given purified and clean water. They are good water drinkers today because of that.

The formula to determine how much water to drink is based on your weight divided by 2. For example, 160 pounds ÷ 2 = 80 ounces of water. Your body will let you know if you're getting enough or not. Hydration is covered later in more detail.

Upright spine.

If the spine is aligned, the immune system and body are healthier. Don't allow yourself to walk like a duck! This totally misaligns and breaks down the all-important spine. Stand up straight and make sure your posture is accurate. When people slump and don't pay attention to posture, it makes them look older. The more they move like this, the further the spine will break down. Don't get lazy. Straighten up. Put a pep in your step!

When driving a vehicle, make sure you're sitting up tall and straight. Don't allow yourself to scrunch down and slip lower in the seat. To avoid the dreaded humpback, get in the habit of pushing the head directly back and forward, keeping the chin level. When working at a computer for long periods of time, avoid drooping the head. Find ways to keep that head straight!

I spoke with Dr. Lawrence Quell, a holistic chiropractor and quantum field life coach in Denver, Colorado. He suggests the Yoga Breath of Fire technique to help align the spine:

Do not do this if pregnant. Stand up straight. Put the arms and hands directly over the head. For men, put the right thumb over the left thumb. For woman, put the left thumb over the right thumb. Face palms forward and quickly breathe in. Forcibly breathe out through the nose. You should feel the lower abdomen pushing in and out. The inhale should be soft and the exhale should be loud, but in equal lengths. Do this for at least 30 seconds. Increase the time as you become more comfortable.

Stretch, exercise, go for walks and move the body so the spine stays strong and straight. The immune system is directly connected to the spine, so it makes sense to take good care of it.

Oops!

Be realistic. An unhealthy (but tasty) *carboplunk* can be amazing on occasion, and you should enjoy it to the max! However, repeating this day after day can lead to indulgences which can undermine your progress. Don't let the addiction reclaim its lost territory. Enjoy once, then let go and return to your goal.

Choose nutrition and embrace this new lifestyle. Don't

argue with it. Decide NOW on conscious nutritional intake with realistic flexibility and adaptability. Choose your poisons carefully.

Wealth of a treat.

Years ago, I read a book about a politician's daughter who was kidnapped and whisked away to the Columbian jungle. For several years in captivity, she survived on what little food was provided, most lacking any nutritional benefits. Her captors were attempting to gain money and political power from her relatives and connections, so she was treated slightly better than other abductees. When she was finally able to resume her life, her biggest pleasure was to go to the grocery store and purchase nutritious items like fresh fruits and vegetables. After so many years, these were treats for her.

It is a gift to have a selection of quality and nutritious items. Salty, fatty and sugary items are not treats. The body wants and needs nutrition that is both physically and energetically nourishing. It is a great prosperity to have so many healthy choices.

Divine nutrition.

Whether plant or animal based, each organism has given its life for our human consumption. This relationship deserves appreciation, gratefulness and respect. I thank and bless with love everything I put into my mouth. It is proven that molecules align in divine geometric patterns when meditation, positive visualization and prayer are used. There are several noted studies in this area, including those of Massaru

Emoto[15]. When divine geometric patterns are in place, nutrients are more easily absorbed. It is also 90% energy. Energy feeds energy. It either nourishes or is hollow and empty.

Everyone who handles a food item leaves behind a bit of energy called an imprint. Their negativity or love in that moment has an impact. Blessing what we eat can also remove previous negative energy, replacing that space with gratefulness and appreciation. This enhances energetic nutrition.

On my water filter container, I write the words *Love*, *Hydration* and *Health* so I do not have to bless every single glass. This way, the words provide their healthy vibration and will never be forgotten or overlooked. When I bless my food, I thank it for giving up its life or part of its life to sustain my own. Keep it simple and straightforward. It does not have to be seriously heavy, fancy or lengthy. It is a personal choice. The intent is what makes it work.

This type of approach connects us to what we are consuming and can aid in making better choices. It's gratitude in being aware. It is a means of being consistently and lovingly connected. When divine geometry is involved, it's an opportunity to connect with both physical and spiritual nutrition.

These concepts help a person make better choices, be a more tuned-in listener, and avidly support the body. Refrain from judging yourself so harshly. Get lovingly reconnected with your body. When it realizes it is being listened to, it will speak up more often and more clearly. It will be easier to know what, how and when to do exactly what you need to do.

---

15 Masaru Emoto's book,"The Hidden Messages in Water," 2004, Wikipedia, https://en.wikipedia.org/wiki/Masaru_Emoto

Meditation and prayer.

There are several forms of meditation. In meditation, the mind is cleared of thought. It is focused attention with a quiet mind. You can use visualization, music, guided or self-paced. Meditation is a way to direct your thoughts and body toward love, compassion, gratitude, joy and kindness. When fear, negativity and worry arise, just take note and move them along. Bring yourself back to your quiet inner being. Let go of any comparisons. Gain insight with the self and spirit, set an intention, and align emotion with the mind. In this focused state, the body and mind can heal. I am fond of Dr. Joe Dispenza's work on this subject.

Prayer is highly personal and very effective. Be grateful and thank the higher being for the abundance you desire. When you ask for something, it's fine to expect results, but don't demand them. Believe it will happen in the right time. Spirit knows.

Please note that wishing harm, blame or harsh judgment on another will only hurt you. If this is tempting to you, seek out different ways of thinking and heal yourself. Prayer is meant for insight, growth, guidance, peace and healing.

Reclaim your power.

You are meant to think, feel, laugh and create, but this confused society has most everyone believing and living otherwise. I firmly believe these concepts come full circle. Energy knows when it is being supported, and this impacts what is being attracted. It may seem small, but it has an impact on life now and in the future.

There are energetic and physical disruptions that must be

considered. Turn off the shallow, narrow-minded television and other technology. Too much of this noise clutters the mind, manipulates thinking and seriously limits our views. It also disrupts healthy digestion. Build a broader awareness of life. Connect with nutrition, the earth, the cosmos, the heart and the Divine. Create. When we create, these efforts impact energetic geometrical patterns. Sing or dance while preparing food. Joy makes the experience a lot more fun!

If a belief about nutrition is based in a negative emotion such as fear, shame or guilt, then find a way to think differently. This is why it is necessary to reboot, reclaim and refocus nutrition. All things must be approached with individual wisdom. Live wiser. Seek truth directly from within, from the source. This trusting relationship is developed over time. Human beings are meant to go through their own unique discovery and acceptance processes. Gain better understanding of those processes which result in soul enlightenment.

We have been taught how to think and act when it comes to food, especially through peer pressure. I once saw my daughter-in-law hand half an avocado to my grandson with a spoon. He gobbled it down without adding a thing. It was gorgeous and gratifying to watch. We learn from each other, especially those who dare to think outside the socially-designed cage that inhibits our natural ability for discernment. It opens our minds to new ideas that can better serve us and our bodily needs. We help each other, we need each other, and we need you!

Refocus intent.

Set a healthy intent every day. Follow and to listen to it, and consciously be determined to take care of this precious body. Don't get out of bed until you have taken on the right attitude and set the day's intention. Whatever the size or shape, this body requires respect and love. Give it what it needs.

When setting intent for the day, give this technique a try:

Close your eyes, look to the left and say to yourself, "Engage the left brain." Next, look to the right and say, "Engage the right brain." Look forward toward the bridge of the nose and say, "Both sides of my brain are engaged and working together. My intent for today is______."

This is what happens when a person is channeling or having a psychic moment. Both sides of the brain are engaged. Do not walk around in this state for long periods; it is not normal for most humans. This is an old technique that works. When you do this, you are likely to feel a slight buzz in the head because it is different from how your brain has been trained to function.

Usually, one side of the brain is more dominant than the other at any given time. The left is more logical, while the right is the more creative side. If you look at images of Einstein's brain you will see there is not much distance between the right and left hemispheres. Those of us with more common brains have a clear and distinct distance. It is possible to lessen this distance, so it makes sense to strive for it and get both sides working together. Be careful, though. Walking around all day with both sides engaged is overloading. Psychics who stay in this state too long can cause real health issues with the brain. The brain needs rest from such things. Our brain has evolved the way it has for a reason. Keep everything in healthy balance.

We are meant to be out of balance from time to time. Falling in love or winning at something are examples of emotion and energy being out of balance. If we remain too long, energy will try to naturally balance things. Ever notice when you are in a heightened and excited state how the rug can suddenly get pulled out? Enjoy the moment, then calm yourself and recenter. This also regains necessary and healthy humility.

To be.

Get to know who you are. Face yourself honestly, realistically, without judgment, and become your own creation. You are always your harshest critic. Making mistakes are part of growth, so you must let go of being overly cruel toward yourself. Stepping up and surpassing these hindrances is true growth. You may have heard that if you want great friends, you must be a great friend. If you want to be around people with integrity, then you must BE that kind of person. Recognizing those who have little or no integrity can be helpful. Whether they see it in themselves or not, they want to be associated with those who do. It can help them look and feel better. Become educated and aware so these people are not able to undermine so easily. Study some of the more positive archetypes and other challenging personalities.

Archetypes are the different parts of our personality. All have *positive* and *shadow* effects. It can be most helpful for recognizing personality pitfalls within your own approach to life. Everyone has a combination of many archetypes. It is not your place to be judgmental or try and diagnose someone; stay in your own life lane. Learning about the more challenging personality types can aid in recognizing them. They are everywhere.

To have a general idea of any subject, it is best to read at least five books on that subject. This may sound like a lot, but one or two books cannot give sufficient information toward understanding or avoiding pitfalls. Remember that you are simply developing an awareness, so leave the diagnosing to professionals.

Back to the reboot.

Rebooting is an action. Observing when, where and why we eat can clue you into inner and outer influences. Write down when, why and how you eat. Keep track of any emotions that rise up. This action can aid in discovering areas of thinking that can be improved. There are many lists available to choose from. Seek one out that makes sense to you.

The written word has profound vibrations, so write down healthier options such as going for a walk or having a warm cup of something healthy, even if it's just hot water. When we recognize what triggers us to consume questionable items, we face truth. If you always have a second glass of wine after the first, try starting with a non-alcoholic drink next time. There are many options.

Once, I was with a dear friend at a bar. I wanted something yummy and refreshing, but not alcoholic. I ordered a lemonade (not really healthy, but refreshing). To me, this is an amazing dessert beverage. My friend informed me that because I was in a bar I should order an alcoholic drink. I laughed and simply mentioned that this was my beverage of choice.

Do not allow others to pressure you. Change takes consistency, persistence, patience, time and creativity. If something is important, people will find a way. You do not live by accident but with intention and self-acceptance. Be what you can accept. Let go of any victim mentality, as this only weakens you and makes you vulnerable to outside influences. Don't escape through food and beverages. Nutrition, nutrition, nutrition.

When a person is truly determined to achieve something, all efforts, actions and thoughts go in that direction. Life pulls in many directions, so please do not give up.

Healthy vibrations.

Refocus to become what we love! It's natural to take care of our body with respect, appreciation, consistency, loyalty and gratitude. In return, communication becomes clearer with the body and the Divine. It is a means to reconnect to the life-giving source which reminds us there is much more to us than we could ever imagine. This is also based in quantum physics[16]. Albert Einstein once said that reality is merely an illusion, although a very persistent one. We have the power to view reality in a healthy and supportive way. When it comes to nutrition, weigh the facts and learn the tricks to helping you understand what the body wants and does not want. Learn about communication and guidance in your body's energetic field and beyond. It is a lost art for many. It's time to regain this precious skill.

---

16 Cate Montana, M.A., "The Illusion of Reality: The Scientific Proof That Everything is Energy and Reality Isn't Real," January 2017, ConsciousLifestyle Magazine excerpt from The E-Word: Ego, Enlightenment & Other Essentials, https://www.consciouslifestylemag.com/everything-is-energy-illusion-reality/

Getting in touch with those subtle and gentle vibrations opens communication channels on deeper levels. These small shifts can be defined. It is a skill most all have within themselves; it is labeled as intuition. Perhaps you've seen a small child who happened to be very focused on something in her hands. She wandered around with it, not really paying attention to the room, yet on occasion she would avoid an obstacle on the floor even though she may not have seen it directly. There was a denser energy the child felt around the object, so she automatically adjusted by lifting her foot over it. Unfortunately, children lose many of these sensitive skills by age four. How different the world might be if this sensitivity was fostered instead of inhibited.

There are many energy-based healing arts and modalities. Sound, color, light, Qi Gong, Tai Chi, hypnotherapy, laying on of hands, meditation, mudras and Reiki are my most favorite. I have taught Reiki (an ancient art of manipulating, clearing and balancing energy with itself and the physical body) for many years. What they all have in common is the ability to connect to the "white spark of life" within. This is the communication and healing center we all have access to.

As with all things, even among the healing arts there can be misinformation and corruption. One in particular teaches that people can suck knowledge right out of you at will. I once had a student who was trained in this art. Because of this belief, she was the only Reiki student I refused to train at the Master-Teacher level. She firmly believed that others were after her knowledge and that there was no way she could keep them from stealing it energetically. She wanted to stop them so they would be forced to pay money for it. Worrying about people not paying for energetic communication is a disastrous misinterpretation and is based in false ego.

Energy is always communicating with other energy. Have you ever been at a party where one negative person walks in and the whole room gets heavy? It can change the whole atmosphere if we allow it. We choose what is allowed in and out!

Religions of all kinds support these concepts. In the laying on of hands, for example, a healer places his hands on someone's crown chakra. He vibrates his hands at a specific number of vibrations per minute while using words, thoughts and actions to tap into the divine spiritual healing realm—often with the help of unseen beings like angels, guides and ancestors. Healing techniques like this have been around for thousands of years. They are not specific to any gender, nationality, culture or belief system. In fact, most who practice the laying on of hands are not trained beyond this technique. It is still influential, regardless.

In Western science, observation is mainly based on seeing an object in a space independent of the person observing it. This is somewhat contradicted by the study of geometric patterns which form through prayer and meditation. I love science. It all has great value. To see the measurable vibration of a food is wonderful! There are many areas of Western science that confirm energetic approaches. For example, when a baby has a buildup of bilirubin in the system, doctors use a blue light to aid the liver in getting rid of excess bilirubin. The blue frequency balances the vibration of the liver while the light warms and increases circulation. This procedure is actually a form of color and light therapy. Scientists have measured the effects of color and sound vibration on people. It is extremely valuable knowledge.

Eastern arts and sciences have studied the energy system in detail and at great length. The human body has 114 chakras and 72,000 nadis, which represent energetic communication points throughout the body. Some are small, some medium and some large. Together, they form a cone-like coil. The narrow end faces and enters the body. The cone elongates and contracts, widens and narrows depending on the energetic health it supports. Energy travels in and out with ease. Chakras bring in and send out energetic information. It is a process that cannot be stopped. You can choose what comes in and out by the way you think and live. Many techniques are available to aid in self-protection from negative energy.

Many in the energetic fields choose to focus on the 7 main chakras. When learning Reiki, I was told by my celestial team to include the ear chakras, so I have ever since. These 8 chakras are influenced by tones and sounds, words, thoughts, colors, intentions, light and other vibrations in the world. Each of the main chakras affects the health of certain organs, systems in the body and our thinking. Eastern philosophies have a vast knowledge about our energy body. When the energy is imbalanced, disrupted or the like, it affects every aspect of our being. When energy is in balance, the vibration becomes healthy and aligns the unhealthy areas of the physical body.

Chakra Awareness Chart

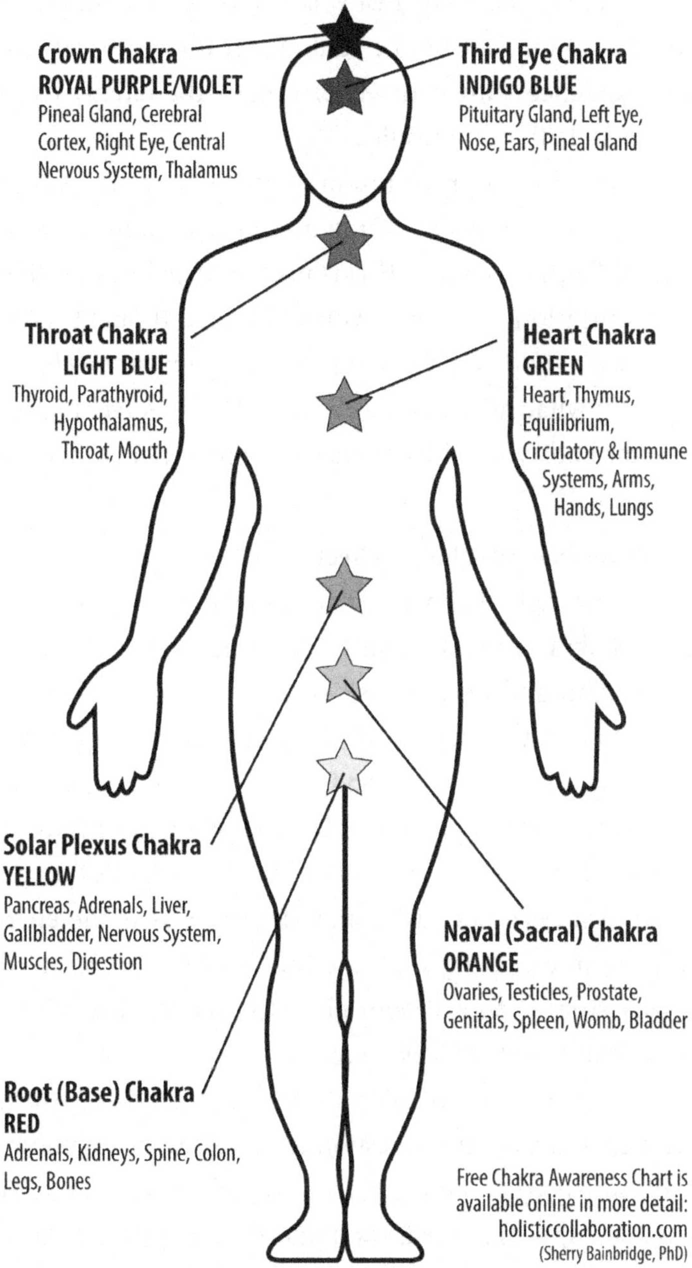

The focus of this book is on eating healthier and learning to listen to the body. Below is a common technique that can be used for this, but be cautious. If there is great stress or fraudulence with yourself or others, the energy can be skewed and affect the results.

Always use your common sense. Use your eyesight, heart and brain together. Only use this technique on yourself, NOT other people. This is just another form of divine communication. At times, you may have thought, *Something is wrong. I can feel it in the pit of my stomach!* This is exactly what might be happening. Use this technique to show the body you are listening to its guidance in nutritional decisions:

The Navel (Sacral) chakra check.

Place your right palm an inch away from and over the sacral chakra, which is slightly above the belly button. Feel its vibration and its size. Ask your body if it wants potato chips. Notice the energy recoiling inward, getting tighter and smaller. Now ask your body if it wants an organic apple. Notice the chakra opening wider, feeling lighter inside and just outside the body. Can you feel it? Practice this for yourself until it becomes easier and clearer. This is the energy body communicating through and with the physical. The grocery store is an excellent place to practice this, as there are so many food choices there.

The easiest way to calibrate for accuracy is to ask the sacral chakra a control question for an answer you know to be absolutely true. If it recoils inward, which feels dense and heavy as it spirals towards the spine, the energy is backwards and needs to be reset. This can be done by calming down and using rhythmic breathing. Inhale and hold for a moment, then exhale and hold for a moment. Repeat this twice more. You can also hydrate with water. Prayer, meditation, connecting with source and grounding with mother earth are all excellent ways to rebalance and reset the energy.

Keep this fun! Don't make it serious. It can help when done accurately. Use it to support and give guidance to change. If it's not joyful, it won't last. Be grateful for such a lovely technique and give it time to develop. For some, it can be hard at first to feel the energetic movement. Don't pressure yourself. Keep it light and natural, because it is.

Silly permission, or is it?

You must give yourself permission to be healthy and to be connected with the body. It is your own best communication instrument. It simply needs to be rediscovered and utilized. Like a muscle, it needs to develop strength. Remember, you are the one who has taught your body over time. Explain to it what you are doing. The more positive you make your experience, the more sustaining the change will be. Einstein once said, "There are only two ways to live your life. One is as though nothing is a miracle. The other is as though everything is a miracle." It is truly a miracle that your body has survived what you have put it through thus far. The relationship between the physical and spiritual is miraculous!

The need to be flexible and adaptable in our thinking is ever-changing. Even science recognizes this. Over time, what it thought it knew before has now proven wrong. As smaller and smaller particles are discovered, new knowledge comes to light. If the body decides that one type of food is no longer desired, our thinking must change so better actions may follow. Nothing stays the same in energetic or physical life. All is ever expanding and evolving. Learning to listen to the body is the most powerful thing a human can do toward health and well-being. In fact, this way of thinking can bring back the fun. Food begins to take a more appropriate place, as it will no longer be the main focus in life. This can be an adventurous, pleasurable and supportive approach.

Eating is an opportunity to connect with others. Slow down, set aside technology and connect, or just be silent as you nourish and hydrate. Be mindful and aware. It's all nourishment for the body and soul.

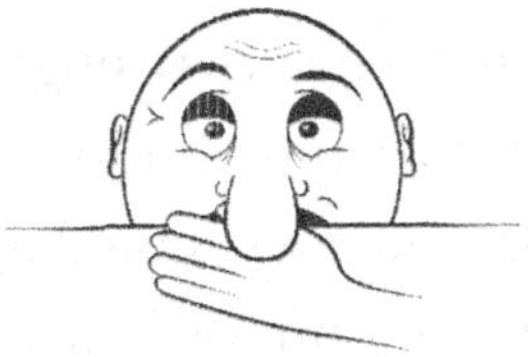

3| Digestive Communication

When the chest cavity gets full of fat, it has no other place to go but outward; the upper stomach begins to protrude. Those with barrel chests naturally have more room to accommodate it (it naturally protrudes a bit), but it's a sign to reevaluate what is being eaten. We don't want the precious organs being packed in fat, which can constrict everything around it.

The best communication we have with our consumption is the digestive system. It takes a lot of energy to digest, which is why bland diets are recommended when a person is ill. To aid the digestive system during ailments, lightly cook all fruits and vegetables and avoid heavy meats and alcoholic beverages. If the body temperature rises when eating, the body is dampened. This is a Chinese term that means the digestive system is stressing the body and needs to be treated easier. This can happen in times of heavy stress or when the body indicates an underlying issue. Support this valuable system by being aware of it.

Study the internal organs and what they do. Knowing where the organs are located, along with their functions, is helpful for many reasons. Understanding how systems work can aid in asking better questions. Learn about the physical body *before* something goes wrong. You need a general understanding from hormones to toenails. Learn how different parts can work individually and together. Take a class or read a book. You will gain wisdom and patience with the body.

Pay attention to any sensations inside or outside the body—poop, urine, mucous, etc. **Please be sure to check with your doctors and/or nutritional experts.** Since most Western doctors have no education in nutrition, seeking out professional alternative advice can be advantageous. Self-diagnosing can be informative, but it also can be harmful. These are only a few things to consider when learning to listen to what the body is saying. You have an opportunity to improve what you consume before seeking out prescription medications.

Digestion

Acid reflux.

This occurs when stomach acid travels upward through the esophagus. When swallowing, the sphincter in the throat relaxes to allow food to move to the stomach. It does not fully close, leaving a gap that can allow acid to get through. Acid tastes sour or bitter in the mouth and can make the throat feel sore. It can also cause a burning sensation in the chest and is damaging. Get it checked out by a proper professional to rule out any other underlying issues.

There are other options. For example, vinegar is a pH

reducer, which means it increases acid. It has many benefits, but the more it processes the less value it can provide. If you do not like the taste of vinegar, your body is likely saying it is not the correct choice. Working with a professional usually provides several alternatives.

Acid reflux can also indicate a lack of hydrochloric acid in the stomach. To compensate for this, the body produces more. Taking antacids for reflux can actually cause the stomach to overcompensate. Hydrochloric acid is an option to antacid products and can be purchased in its own form. Follow the directions carefully. It generally requires a bit of experimenting by taking one capsule initially before eating. More capsules can be added until relief occurs.

Reflux can also be a sign that the body does not like what is being consumed; or, on the mental side, there may be too much worry or stress. Some foods may be inherently acidic or spicy. As the body changes over time, these can be warnings that something needs to be modified. Food enzymes and hypnotherapy are also good alternatives.

If the body is too acidic, take steps to make it more alkaline. This will help the body at all levels. Get rid of preprocessed foods and sugars, limit red meats and increase colorful vegetables and fruits. Stay well-hydrated, and try some green tea once in a while. Avoid lying flat after eating. Sometimes a bit of sugar-free (natural) gum after eating can help keep the acid down in the stomach.

Citrus.

Citrus (except lemons and limes) will be the last to digest if eaten along with food. It must be eaten separately at least

20 minutes before and after anything else. In the stomach, citrus juices will back up through any food, creating a frothy mess which causes the digestive system to push it through more quickly. Less nutrients are absorbed this way. Citrus is an acid. Lemons and limes are assimilated as alkaline into the body, which is helpful. Make sure that the teeth and mouth are thoroughly cleaned 20 minutes after eating these. The teeth can be harmed by rubbing the acid into the enamel with a toothbrush, so allow the saliva to do its job first.

Eating.

Slow down and chew smaller bites. Keep track of the food combinations and note any symptoms that arise. Do not eat if coughing and try using a humidifier if the throat seems dry. Stay hydrated so that eating does not involve loading glasses of water into the system; this only stretches the stomach. Keep the stomach at a healthy size. One fad diet recommended loading a glass or two of water before eating, then more while eating to make a person feel fuller. The goal should be to shrink the stomach. Too much liquid is hard on the body and raises blood pressure. Use the eyes to determine the proper amount to eat.

Notice the thinking that underlies the eating. During vacation, many people throw caution to the wind and consume all the things they have been avoiding. That's sabotage! You can still have fun and eat healthy while on vacation. Have a treat or two, but coming home 10+ pounds heavier does not make sense. I make it a game to lose a little weight on vacation by eating healthy with limited treats (choose your poisons carefully). There is no need to deprive yourself of anything, though. It's all a matter of how a person chooses to look at it.

Chew slowly so the saliva has time to do its job. Gulping food is ridiculous and potentially harmful. A person I knew would take such big bites that he had to push his head forward like a turtle to even swallow. It was painful to watch. Plopping large portions into the stomach can easily cause the acid to increase so it can deal with the onslaught. It is neither impressive nor attractive to take giant bites of anything. Smaller bites reduce stress on the esophagus and help the stomach metabolize the food. It allows the digestive enzymes in the saliva to work better. This also helps alleviate bloating and helps with weight loss. Eating slower creates a better hormonal response from the body, makes digestion easier, helps strengthen the bones in the mouth and teeth, increases body energy, and is simply more enjoyable.

Flour and processed foods.

Pulverized items are like sugars to the body. Flour products get absorbed in the upper stomach because they are so easily digested. This increases insulin and spikes the glucose. Each body has a specific number of spikes that occur before their threshold for diabetes risk is reached.

Non-pulverized, cooked brown rice does not completely break down as it travels through the stomach, but breaks down more in the intestinal tract. Nutrients are absorbed at each stage, and the intestinal lining also gets cleaned. If it is pulverized, it gets absorbed too early, bypassing its many benefits and nutrients. Eating things closer to their natural state is nature's way.

Gas and bloating:.

Intestinal gas is normal. The average person can produce as much as three pounds per day. Carbon dioxide, hydrogen and methane (for some) mix with nitrogen and oxygen from the air we breathe or swallow to create a bacterium that forms the gas. If the gas has an unpleasant odor, this is a warning sign that something is not right. Normal gas does not stink. Other reasons for gas might be swallowing too much air, not chewing correctly, taking large bites, drinking carbonated beverages, gulping beverages, overeating, constipation, illness, certain medications, too many starchy foods (bread and grains), too much fat, or even gluten sensitivity.

Intestinal tract.

Each stage of the digestive system has its job of extracting nutrients. Processed foods are a problem because they do not allow for natural processing. Putrefied feces can build up on the walls of the intestines. This causes the parasites that naturally live within us to multiply, putting things out of balance. It also affects the lining's ability to absorb nutrients. Brown rice is an excellent way to help clean this out. If needed, the Psyllium Husk detoxifying recipe *[see next section]* can be used over a 10 to 20-day period to clean this out. A doctor can also order a strong laxative that will do the same job.

The digestive system needs the proper space in which to work. When fat builds up around the tract, it causes all sorts of problems. A twisted or squished tract is serious. Give it the room it needs. Too much fat built up in the small intestines can cause chronic diarrhea, coat the lining of the intestines, and even lead to malnutrition.

Liver.

This important digestive organ can get overloaded with toxins. When this happens, the liver dispels them into the bloodstream for the kidneys to handle. If they are more than the kidneys can handle, they get secreted out through the lungs and skin. This can cause bad breath and skin odor. This condition overloads the immune system and compromises resistance to illness and disease. Take good care of this organ! Limit alcohol, do not mix alcohol with medications and do not chemically alter drugs or other items. Decrease toxins as much as possible to help the liver stay healthy. This is an amazing organ, but it does have limitations. Don't wait until the liver gets damaged before making a healthier change.

Liquids.

Do not drink large amounts of liquids before, during or after eating. Avoid liquids 15 minutes before eating. Swallow food completely before taking in liquids to ensure that chewing has done its job. Take time to enjoy the senses with food. Spread out liquids evenly during the day. It is recommended to have a few swallows every 20 minutes. This may not be workable, but it helps the body to not have large quantities all at once.

Mucus.

Mucus in the throat can be an early warning of an allergy or food sensitivity such as with dairy, soy, nuts, eggs or shellfish. Avoid foods that cause mucus to form. This could also be a sign of asthma, dysphagia or acid reflux. Avoiding foods that contain sulfites (beers, wines, commercially dried fruits, pickled onions, soft drinks) may help.

Blood tests can easily reveal sensitivities and allergies; however, they are not always perfect. Some people who are sensitive to gluten and have all the symptoms of celiac have been known to not show a problem. I have a friend like this. I can tell when she has eaten something with gluten in it. Her face becomes pale, her words get mixed and she struggles to say what she is thinking (foggy-headedness), and she becomes very quiet. When she avoids all gluten, these things do not occur.

Probiotics and enzymes.

If the digestive system is in balance, additional probiotics and enzymes are unnecessary. My body will not allow me to take these. I will get diarrhea every time. This has shocked many people because they cannot understand that each body is different. Mine apparently does not need any extra.

Sweat.

When a person is drinking and eating healthy, sweat can actually smell sweet and is rarely unpleasant. It is the body's way of getting rid of hormones and toxins. It cools down an overheated body. This part of the digestive system can easily be overlooked. Emotions (such as anger), exercise, stress, disease/illness, body heat, caffeine, toxins, hot or spicy foods, hot beverages, alcohol, medications, heart rate, blood pressure, hormones and pregnancy all affect sweating. It can be an early indication of an imbalance with the body, diet, environment and/or thinking.

Avoid products that contain harmful ingredients like aluminum, which is commonly used in deodorant. In research, there is much controversy, but there is some evidence of its link to neurodegenerative disease and more. Aluminum will absorb through capillaries in the skin and, in my opinion, build up over time. This requires individual consideration, research and wisdom. I rarely use an aluminum-based antiperspirant. When I choose to, it is natural and coconut oil-based. It works for me, but may not for others. Talk to professionals and check out other countries' approaches. Notice any emotions that rise when sweat is triggered. A simple change in thinking can be effective. This is highly personal and diverse. Limit aluminum intake as much as possible. Excessive sweating can be an indication of a much more serious underlying issue.

Waste/poop.

This is one of the best ways to measure health. Feces (poop) are the waste products being eliminated from the body. Each person has different types. Some have looser stools, different shapes, colors, and levels of smells. Poop should pass easily with very little strain. Blood in the waste, which can cause the poop to be black, is serious and needs the opinion of a medical professional. Red, black, green, yellow or white poop can indicate a possibly serious condition, and a professional opinion should be sought out immediately. Certain foods can also affect the color. Any significant change from the norm can indicate a more serious issue. Take the time to look at it and to be aware of what is normal and healthy.

In general, poop should not have a horrific odor. It should sink to the bottom of the toilet. If it floats, it's most likely full of fat. If it contains chunks of food, then chew the food longer. Some foods such as corn are not digestible, so there will always be kernels showing. Stools should be medium to dark in color, which indicates a person is usually eating dark leafy greens and vegetables. Strong stool odors and gas can indicate an imbalance in bacteria or eating unhealthy and highly processed items. Those should be passed in a single piece or a few smaller pieces. Stools should be passed one to three times a day. Some can even pass up to five times on certain days, depending on an individual's own digestive system and what is being eaten.

Frequency can also vary based on what is being consumed, medications being taken, hydration levels, fiber-richness of foods, amount of exercise, depression, thyroid health, nervous system issues, and even stress levels. The Bristal stool chart can easily be located on the Internet. It's a great guide to what is normal for most. The human body can hold up to 7-60+ pounds of waste. The longer the feces sit in the intestines, the more putrefied they can become.

A proper digestive system is essential. It is an indication of health and a balanced diet. Abnormalities that last longer than a couple of weeks can indicate a more serious issue and can lead to complications. Ongoing diarrhea affects nutrition, while constipation can lead to obstructions in the intestinal tract, both of which are serious. Poop talks! Know this part of the body, look at it, research and talk to doctors. Learn what is normal and what indicates abnormal.

There are many reasons a person may not eliminate properly. Do NOT be tempted to use laxatives on a regular basis. The idea is to determine the real cause and to solve it. Find out the specific reason, whether it's physical, mental, emotional, spiritual or environmental. Be determined to uncover the root cause.

Urine.

Urine ranges from clear to a pale-yellow color. Changes in color, odor, comfort and ease of passing can all indicate a problem. Brown urine denotes dehydration and lack of electrolytes, which can often be resolved with over-the-counter solutions. In severe cases, medical attention should be sought immediately. Some foods such as beans, blackberries and those with vitamins A and B can darken urine. Hydration level, medications, liver issues, infection or disease can affect the darkness, so check with professionals if this occurs. Pink or red urine can also indicate a more serious issue that should be checked out immediately.

Urine should be excreted without pain and in a steady stream. It should not require force, as this can cause damage to the urethra (inner tube). Pain or interrupted flow can indicate an issue that should be checked out by a physician immediately.

A person generally pees 6-7 times per day, but 4-10 times per day is not unusual. Age, bladder size, hydration, medical conditions, hormonal changes, pressure on the bladder (pregnancy or fat), amount of alcohol, drugs, medications, caffeine and supplements can all affect frequency. About 64 ounces (1/2 gallon) of fluid per day is generally recommended. The body is 70% water; it is basic to our health.

Peeing too often or not enough, having back pain, odd color, fever, leakage, pain or a strong odor are all indications there might be an issue that should be checked out, especially if any are dramatic. Detecting something early makes it easier to deal with. It is not uncommon for people to have some leakage as they age, cough, sneeze or laugh hard. This can especially happen with women, due to how short the tube is. Strengthen the muscles in the lower abdomen and see if this improves.

Dehydration or consuming extra liquids affects how often and how much a person urinates; but be aware that dehydration followed by quick rehydration is not healthy. Hydrate slowly. When people are in serious situations (such as being lost and having gone without hydration), never hydrate quickly. It can have serious affects by lowering sodium in the blood to dangerous levels. Overnight urination should not occur more than 1-2 times. If more often, speak to a trusted physician or specialist. Many things can affect how often a person gets up to pee during the night. If you exercise more during the day, you are likely to get up throughout the night. Conversely, if you don't get good exercise, you may not get up often overnight. Lifestyle choices and body fluids also affect the frequency of getting up during the night.

Do not cut back on healthy consumption just to pee less often. If night urination is an issue and doctors cannot determine the cause, just drink earlier in the day and avoid drinking in the evening.

Electricity travels faster in water. Energy/spirit can communicate easier if the body is well-hydrated. Doing any energetic or spiritual work will dehydrate the body. People often get dehydrated after being in church, giving a meaningful speech, aiding others in healing, having a parenting moment, doing intuitive work or physical therapy.

Consider keeping a journal to track what is normal and not normal. It can be most helpful in picking up on patterns, like how specific foods or liquids affect digestion or sleep.

Notice any digestive complaints such as foggy-headed thinking, rapid weight gain or loss, gas, bloating, belching, hiccups, abdominal aches, itching in the mouth or throat, stuffiness, mucus, headache, coughing or dry throat. These are signs that the body is having a problem with the nutrition level, the combination of food or the amount and type of beverages. Each person is different, so one must do this according to his or her own body.

The digestive system is a major regulator to health. As a person ages, the system will indicate changes in diet to keep the body in balance. For example, if a negative change occurs in the digestive system after eating spicy foods, then lessen the level of spice. The body will step up to help when it feels listened to, valued, loved and supported.

The physical body speaks beyond the digestive system. When I get a pimple or boil on my right shoulder blade, it is an indication that illness is not far behind. When another one shows up directly across on the other shoulder blade, I know I need to seek medical attention because something is wrong. I immediately take extra care of myself through diet, lessening my stress and properly hydrating.

Leg cramps are usually due to low calcium, while others may find they are low in potassium. When my right big toe aches, I know it's a sign of stress and/or lack of hydration, which could make my body vulnerable to cancer. Dehydration also raises my blood pressure and thickens my blood. Learn to connect intuition with the physical. The body can show certain indicators before actually coming down with symptoms.

I make my own body oils. When I learned that sesame oil is one of the closest oils to the sebum (skin oil), I began to use sesame oil as a carrier (base) in the mixture. Using it on my face caused a skin infection which required a prescription cream to keep my face from breaking out. I had caused my skin to think it had too much sebum, so it reacted. I now rotate my base oils so they are not consistently used over time. The body requires variety. I also use organic cleanser and moisturizer on my face, leaving this to professionals who are more skilled than me.

Ask questions about everything. For example, lavender oil can cause a woman to go into labor in the first and last trimesters. All things have side effects (contraindications). Herbs and essential oils are no different than medications. Consistent use of one product over time can be as damaging as pharmaceuticals. Too much of anything creates an imbalance. Extremes are not healthy.

There is a Law of Similarity for medicinal plants, and it's how our ancestors knew which plants to use for certain maladies. For example, if a consumed plant caused a horrific headache, a small amount would then be administered to relieve the headache. If one caused vomiting, a small amount of that plant would be eaten afterward. Nature is amazing! I do not recommend going around testing plants, as that could be potentially deadly. Use available resources, ask questions and speak to knowledgeable people directly.

It is so important to get in tune with energy and the body and to find out what is unique in their communications.

What works for one may very well be harmful to another. I can share my education and experiences along with my clients' experiences. People must still decide for themselves. I am a firm believer in hypnosis. It can identify issues and aid the body in healing. Choose mentors and teachers carefully. Don't just turn your health over to others. Of course, if involved in a crisis, choice is not reasonable; so having trust is likely your best option. There are many excellently trained individuals for such times.

Read the certificates and educational documents that are displayed in professionals' offices. By law, those must be posted. Check with state exam boards and regulators to validate their credentials. While in Arizona, I met a woman who claimed she was a licensed psychologist. Her actions and lifestyle were not conducive to someone who would have had that education. Something did not seem right. When I called the exam boards, they had no record of her. She had never been licensed in that or any other state.

I am sure this falsehood aided her in selling medical insurance, which was how she made money. It gave her credibility, which I am sure clients respected, and made them feel comfortable buying from her. As an older woman in her late 60s, earning a living can be difficult; but defrauding people is simply wrong, and I no longer have any respect for this person. There are many horror stories involving fake surgeons and other false professionals. Always check with the boards and the regulators. They have active and easy-to-use websites for such purposes.

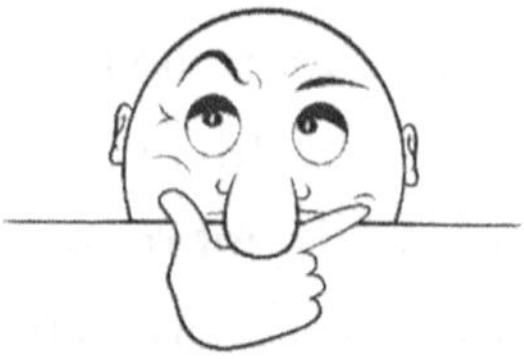

4| Digestion and Elimination

The digestive system is an incredible communicator. It is composed of organs and acids that break down complex food particles into smaller and more absorbable items. There are different stages of digestion, each having its purpose for healthy nutritional support. Every step of digestion has a purpose and absorbs different nutrition from the foods. A whole nut, for example, gets broken down throughout the system before ending up in the intestinal track. Absorption breaks down food to a cellular level so nutrients can be taken in and delivered to where the body needs it most. Digestion requires much energy.

Here are the major organs involved in the digestive and elimination systems (following page):

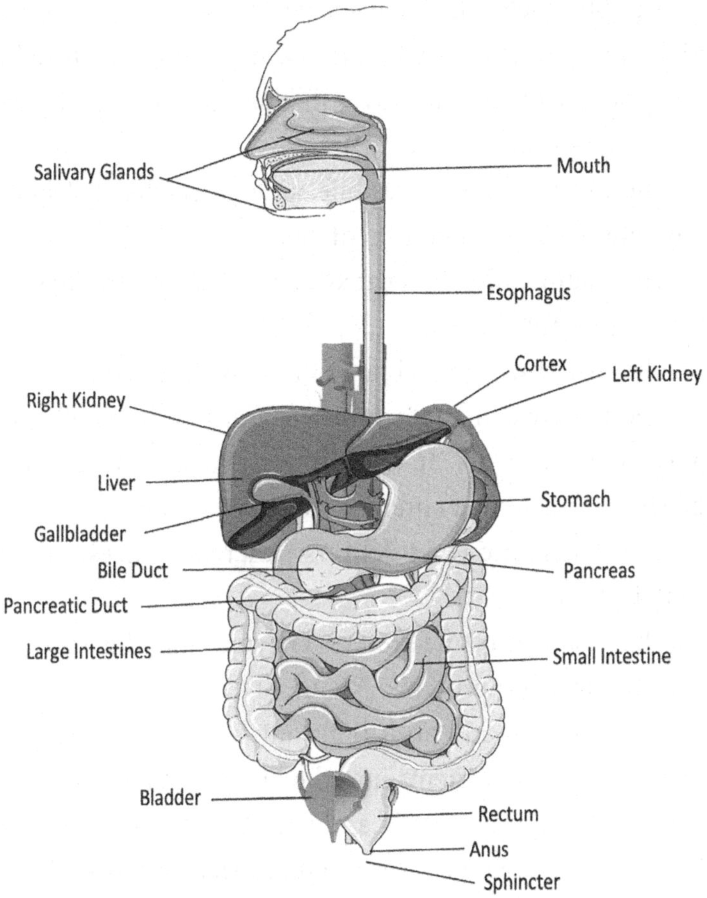

The **Salivary Gland** has a starch-digesting enzyme and a trace of fat-digesting enzyme.

The **Mouth** chews and mixes food with saliva. The teeth are incredibly important as they begin mashing and shredding foods. They aid the saliva in breaking it down so it's more easily digested.

The **Esophagus** passes food to the stomach. Through peristalsis, radially symmetrical muscles move food downward in a wavelike manner via contraction and relaxation.

The **Stomach** adds acid enzymes and fluid. It churns, mixes and grinds food into a liquid mass. Food is stored in the upper part before it moves through the acids and lower part of the stomach.

The **Liver** manufactures bile, a detergent-like substance that helps facilitate digestion of fats.

The **Gallbladder** is located at the base of the liver. It stores bile until needed.

The **Bile Duct** moves bile to the small intestines.

The **Pancreas** manufactures enzymes to digest all energy-causing nutrients. It releases bicarbonate to neutralize the stomach acid that enters the small intestine.

The **Pancreatic Duct** delivers pancreatic juices into the small intestines.

The **Small Intestine** secretes enzymes that digest carbohydrates, fats and proteins. About 20 feet long, it is a major part of digestion and absorbing nutrients. Cells lining the intestine absorb nutrients into the blood and lymph, a fluid composed of lymph vessels and lymph nodes. Lymph flows through the lymphatic system and returns fluid from the tissues to be recirculated.

The **Large Intestine** (Colon) reabsorbs water and minerals. About five feet long, it passes waste, fiber and bacteria, and absorbs any leftover nutrients and water. There are four main parts: cecum, colon, rectum and anal canal. Partially digested food moves through the cecum into the colon, where water, some nutrients and electrolytes are absorbed. Bile does move into the large intestine, but about 90% of the bile salts get reabsorbed into the bloodstream through the small intestine walls. Bile salts must be in balance. Too much can cause diarrhea, trapped gas, bad-smelling gas, stomach cramps, weight loss and/or pale-colored stools.

The **Rectum** stores waste prior to elimination.

The **Anus** holds the rectum closed and opens it to allow elimination.

Kidneys remove waste, toxins and excess water from the blood, then move urine to the bladder. They also make hormones that produce red blood cells and convert vitamin D into its active form so it becomes usable by the body.

The **Cortex** is the outer kidney layer where blood-filtering units (nephrons) begin the blood filtration process. It also creates the hormone erythropoietin, which helps the blood cells and bone marrow.

The **Bladder** is a balloon-like sac that stores urine; it is located in the pelvic area. Urine contains leftover waste and fluids from what the body has taken in. Most adults eliminate from the body about a quart and a half of urine daily.

The **Sphincter** is a circular muscle which maintains constriction until it relaxes (as needed) to eliminate waste.

The stomach and colon have two layers of **Mucus**. The inner layer is attached; the outer layer is not attached and is less dense. Mucus is a habitat for bacteria. Its job is to protect areas from unhealthy bacteria. It clears and separates bacteria from cells that provide physical protection from digestive juices. Mucus helps reduce inflammation and infection.

At each stage, different nutrients are absorbed to provide the body with sufficient energy and molecular building blocks. The digestive system is pretty much the same for all animals. It is miraculous, to say the least.

Chewing and swallowing are part of digestion. When done properly, a person may easily swallow food without swallowing air. If you get gassy after eating, try chewing your food longer and take smaller bites to help the saliva break it down for easier digestion. There are many capillaries in the mouth which are affected by what you put there. Spices, such as cinnamon or peppers, open the capillaries and can activate pain-relieving endorphins. Have you ever noticed that eating can often lessen pain? All attention gets focused on eating, tasting, smelling, hearing and the inherent pleasures they bring.

You are the ruler of your own body universe. There is life upon life within it. When we consume foods, other life forms such as worms and bacteria are also consumed. These unhealthy parasites come from food, water and contact with others, including toilets. Some are considered helpful to the human body, but more research is needed. These are naturally kept in balance by a healthy body. When these become imbalanced, so does your body universe.

The body can hold up to 75 pounds of feces (poop). Over time, feces can attach to the intestinal lining and become putrefied. This type of feces is long, stringy and black. The more putrefied feces there are, the more worms increase in number. They also block important nutrients from being absorbed. Proper elimination is most important. When people lack fiber, eat *carboplunks* (worms love these) or continuously put food into their system while holding feces back from being eliminated, there is no way the intestinal track can keep itself clean.

Below is a recipe for cleaning out putrefied feces from the

small and large intestines. It originated with Edgar Cayce, whose treatments are worth exploring. Since 2005, I have used and recommended this recipe to clients with great success.

Internal Cleansing Recipe

(gentle for upper and lower intestinal tracks)

- ½ Cup Organic Apple or Pear Juice
- 2 Tablespoons Aloe Vera Juice/Gel (Lily of the Desert is mild)
- 2 Tablespoons Chlorophyll (mint flavor is fine) or water with a water soluble
- Super dehydrated fruit and vegetable mix (easily digestible)
- 1 Heaping Teaspoon Psyllium Husk

Pour juice in glass, add the aloe and chlorophyll or mixture, then place a straw in the glass. Add psyllium husk, stir and quickly drink down. If you wait for a minute, it will become as thick as gelatin, which is why you must drink immediately.

- 2 Capsules Cascara Sagrada (tree bark laxative)
- 8 Ounces of Water
- 1 cup Smooth Move Tea (if you feel thick or heavy to help aid things along)

Do the above every night before bedtime for 10-15 days. Drink plenty of water during the day. Keep all ingredients in the refrigerator. After about four days, you are likely to have a day or two of cramping. By the third to fifth day, you are likely to have very long poop lengths. You will see the difference between these putrefied feces and normal ones.

Repeat up to 3 times a year if you feel the need. Otherwise, once every year or two is fine if you have a healthy diet full of fiber.

Alternative Cleansing:

An alternative to the above recipe would be to drink 30 fluid ounces of **Magnesium Citrate** (lemon flavor is good). Follow instructions for a colonoscopy prep from your pharmacy or medical doctor. This involves no food, but clear liquids such as juice and broth are okay. It may be harsh, and you will have diarrhea for 24-48 hours. There is much discomfort and cramping, but it's quicker. Don't be surprised if your doctor chooses different routes when it comes to colonoscopy. An issue with this method is that it's primarily designed to clean the colon more than the small intestines. This is why I prefer to use Cayce's Internal Cleansing Recipe.

IMPORTANT: Always check with your medical professionals for more detailed instructions on using a colonoscopy approach and for approval BEFORE using any alternative approaches!

Slowly add solid foods back into your diet. Choose carefully and avoid *carboplunks*. This is a great opportunity to help your body rebalance and add back low or missing nutrients. You will feel amazing, lighter and healthier.

When the digestive system works properly, it breaks down nutritious items and absorbs nutrients at many different stages. If the body doesn't want certain items, several things can happen such as belching, extra gas, stomach pain, gurgling, diarrhea, constipation, lower back aches, dry skin, sores or rash on skin, unpleasant taste, bad breath, thinning hair, teeth/gum issues, very smelly feces or urine, stomach ache, acid reflux, nausea, foggy head, headaches, sleep issues, gaining weight easily and quickly, and more. All these indicators are clues that the body did not like what you gave it. They could also indicate other issues that should be looked into. With appropriate diagnostics, a medical professional can determine if there are any serious underlying issues.

As a person ages, the body may decide certain foods are no longer desired. Some people love spicy food, but the body lets them know there is a limit to how much can be consumed. It does this by producing excess acid in the stomach and feces which can burn the anus and sphincter when eliminating.

With digestive or skin issues in adults or children, a good way to troubleshoot is to eliminate foods one at a time to discover what a person may be having a problem with. Avoid the suspected food for two weeks, then eat it and see what happens. If any of the above-mentioned symptoms occur, the body is indicating it no longer wants that food.

With some allergies and sensitivities, the medical community can have a tough time figuring out the problem. Not everyone tests as allergic. A close friend of mine has all the symptoms of someone allergic to gluten—foggy head, sleep issues and headaches. She had all the Western tests. Some thought she had multiple sclerosis or other serious diseases. It was hell for her to go through. She decided on her own to remove gluten from her diet. I have watched as she ate something that was supposedly gluten free, but was obviously not. Within minutes, she would turn white, her words would become scrambled and she would become very quiet.

All these symptoms vanished when she completely took gluten out of her diet. She never tested positive for celiac disease or gluten allergy with the Western medicine tests.

As mentioned before, remove the suspected item for a couple of weeks, then eat some of it and see what happens.

Restaurants that offer sensitive and allergy free items tend to serve food that has little to no flavor. Some items on the menu could easily be adjusted to most any allergy. It is lazy to lump them all together, as some restaurants do. Trust can also be an issue. I once watched a waitress pour regular soy sauce into a low-salt soy sauce container. It happens all the time.

It can be daunting to keep track of what you can or can't eat when there is an allergy or sensitivity. Much information is available to help, but it can be overwhelming and confusing. I have a sensitivity to corn which causes me to gain weight extremely quick. Corn is used in many food products, but it may or may not be listed in the ingredients.

Acid reflux is common in many people. Treating it with medicine may be a big mistake. If you lower the acid in the stomach, it reacts by creating more acid. If you try hydrochloric acid, please check with the proper professional to ensure you use this properly. Acid reflux can be caused by not enough natural hydrochloric acid, for which the body will then over-compensate. Stomachs require acid for proper digestion; plunking antacids into them is counterproductive. There are many alternative approaches that can solve many issues without the use of medications.

The skin is usually the last place where problems show up.

By the time you see an indication, the cause is often already present throughout the inner body. Don't ignore the skin!

Hunger tells us that we need nutrition. People can easily get confused and reach for food when they are actually in need of hydration. Craving salty items can mean the body is dehydrated and wants water. Clean water is the body's beverage of choice, but it does have limitations. Drinking too much can flush nutrients from the body and having too little can create a myriad of issues. Find your balance.

The bladder holds urine until it is ready to eliminate. It travels through the urethra (tube) to exit the body at an opening in the penis (men) or in front of the vagina (women). Urine is a great indicator of your hydration level. If it smells bad, you are likely dehydrated. If it is foggy, you should probably get a urine test by your doctor to check the condition of your kidneys. The kidneys flush out toxins and drugs from the blood, release hormones that regulate blood pressure, produce an active form of vitamin D needed for calcium absorption, control the production of red blood cells, and balance body fluids. Do NOT force out your urine! This could damage or collapse the urethra as urine exits the body.

If you have already eaten plenty of food, stop and take notice. It takes time for the body to get a message to the brain that it has had enough food. Also keep an eye on your poop. There are two rules of thumb: If it floats, there is too much fat in your diet; if it's light in color, you are lacking in nutrition. Poop should usually be dark (full of nutrients and vegetables), and sink down (heavy with fiber) in the toilet. If poop is round or marble-like, this indicates a lack of hydration and fiber. People have different types of normal poop.

Some can be well formed and others looser. People poop anywhere from 1-5 times a day. This is based on how, what and when you eat. To make pooping easier, put your feet on a small stool, shift your feet forward onto your toes, or rock slowly from side to side. Poop should always exit easily and need not be forced.

The brain is the boss of the digestive system; they are interdependent. When fear and anxiety are present, the whole body is affected. Stomach acid increases, nerves twitch, and hiccups can occur when these emotions are heightened. Imagine a life where fear doesn't exist, where we stay calm even in extremely challenging situations. This is what alternative professions strive for when working with clients. The whole must be considered. If thinking does not change, health remains the same or worsens.

Digestion takes energy from the body. When sick, eat a bland diet and cook vegetables so they are more easily digested. Take your time eating so you chew properly, enjoying the support these foods provide. Take time to relax for a while after eating to allow digestion to do its work. Do the best you can. Eat earlier in the day to allow digestion to complete by bedtime. The body heals while we sleep.

We are bombarded with how and what to think. Allowing media and mega corporations to tell you how to think gives them the control over your body, mind and wallet. Take control of your own mind. Design your own thinking to work for you and the life you are building. Take back your powerful mind. Many people throughout history have used the brain to heal their bodies and lives. Keep in mind that no single approach will heal everything; it takes a combination of methods.

Adjusting is a way of life. Don't get stuck in beliefs that may not be serving your body and mind. People can become a person of habit and reject all else. Trying new foods, healthy beverages, and herbs expand a person and surprises the body. Many times I have heard people say they will just take a pill and not make any changes. This is detrimental to health and the body's desire to clearly communicate. Alternative approaches have been around for thousands of years compared to Western medicines which has been around just 200 years.

Diagnostics are great, but they aren't perfect. Mistakes and false results are not uncommon. They can help streamline processes, but they are not absolute. Many alternative professionals can test in various ways to help pinpoint an issue. Humans are 90% energy. Everything shows up in the energy and can be discovered before damage to the body can occur. Technology has become more advanced and more sensitive, not only within the medical community but also within alternative medicine.

In holistic work, everything is considered. Relationship with the self, others, work, thinking and the environment all have an effect on the body. Along this route, be sure to verify the credentials of all professionals.

Pay attention to your amazing, incredible, beautiful and ordinary body. Do not wait until serious issues arise. The digestive system is complicated, but it has great communication capabilities. If a person listens to the body and takes action, the body will speak up more loudly and clearly. Pay attention to the sensations in the body during and after eating, as these can clue you into an underlying issue or body concern. This is how you catch potential issues in the early stages. Don't delay. Go to a licensed medical doctor first to get as accurate a diagnosis as possible. Then, you and any other alternative professionals will know exactly what you are dealing with. Diagnosis is where medicine excels. Do not settle for guesses. Get tested first to narrow things down, then you can pinpoint what is going on.

The good bacteria (flora) and quality of the lining are key to keeping it and you healthy. Many chronic metabolic diseases begin in the digestive system. Chronic inflammation is one of the most influential factors. Overall health, exercise, sleep, real nutrition from a variety of whole foods, low stress levels, and plenty of prebiotic fiber keep inflammation down and the digestive system and body healthy.

The digestive and elimination systems deserve respect in both actions and thinking. If you complain because you need to urinate or poop, it tells the body that it's not serving you well. Let these systems tell you when you need to take care of something, then go do it. Always, always wash your hands after eliminating! Many people skip this and thoughtlessly spread disease, illness and bacteria. The body's exit areas are in dark, often moist and warm environments which are perfect for germs to grow. Splashes in the toilet bowl during elimination also splatter on you, the toilet and beyond. Please wash afterward!

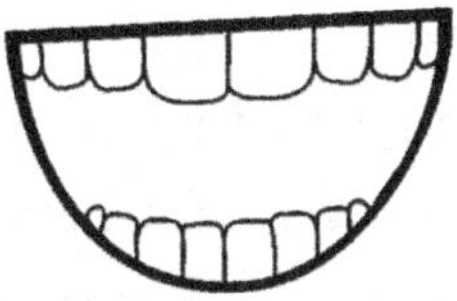

5| Physical Support

One of the biggest pleasures of being a human is our ability to taste and savor flavors. Without the physical body, our energetic form cannot do this. The food industry is highly aware of your love of taste and uses the science of taste, hearing, smelling, seeing and touching to help influence consumers. The more aware we are of this, the better chance we have to choose for ourselves and bypass intentional luring. This is how things are; there is no right or wrong.

The tongue.

One taste bud has 30 to 50 taste receptor (sensory) cells clustered together in bunches, like grapes. There are about 10,000 taste buds on the tongue, the palate and in the throat. Each has hair-like structures called *microvilli* that form a taste pore, a small opening where gasses and particles can pass through the skin.

The food's taste molecules touch the pores and adhere to the hair-like structures. They are then converted into chemical and electrical messages which get sent along the nerves to the brain, where tastes are recognized or labeled. The taste-receptor cells live about 8-12 days, then renew themselves. Smell is a large part of tasting; without it, there is little flavor to anything. Women generally have better smelling ability than men, so their tasting is more sensitive.

Highly processed foods drive people to eat more of the same, resulting in less desire for natural nutrition. *Carboplunks* numb the tongue, causing real food to be less appealing. It is important to give your body time to catch up. Taste buds will return to normal, but they'll need some time. Interestingly, aging causes salt and bitterness sensitivity to reduce faster than savory, sour and sweet.

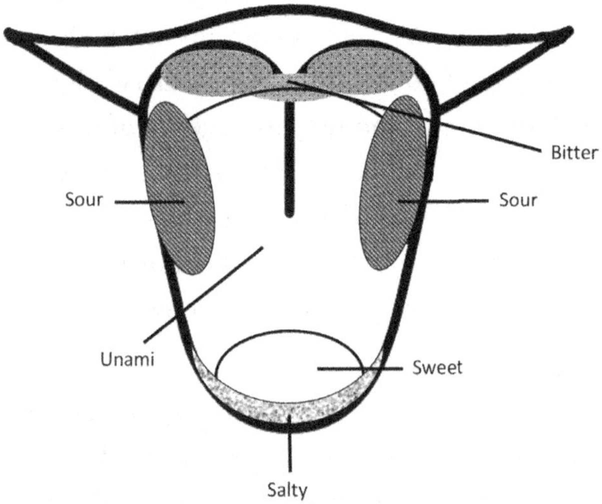

Below are some basic sensory tastes and cravings and what they communicate to the brain. Primaries are in bold.

Bitter (both health-beneficial and dangerous)

- Poisons
- Overripe

- Affects the immune system
- Coffee, leafy greens, raw vegetables, grapefruit, Cacao, radish, oregano, ginger, artichoke, broccoli
- Anti-aging properties
- Improves intestinal flora and balances digestive fluids
- Curbs the desire for sugar

<u>Calcium</u>

- Bitter and chalky
- Vegetables

<u>Cold</u> (cooling sensation)

- Dulls flavor
- Peppermint

Fatty (primary)

- Energy rich
- Brain food

<u>Heat</u> (sensation that affects taste)

- Develops and alters flavor through complex chemical reactions (Maillard reaction) between sugars and certain amino acids. Added spices can alter both flavor and texture when heated.

<u>Metal</u>

- Metallic taste from metal present in food, illness or medications
- Curry, candies, some pastries

Salty (primary)

- Important minerals
- Reduces with age
- Helps to balance electrolytes

<u>Saliva</u>

- Enzymes in the mouth that help to break down the

food and prepare it for digestion
- Aids in tasting dry foods
- Introduces different flavors to taste buds
- Prompts a person to hydrate

Savory or Unami (primary)
- Appetizing proteins
- Tangy, spicy, salty, peppery, seasoned, zesty
- Meats, protein
- Stronger cheeses, condensed foods (tomato paste, etc.), mushrooms

Sour (primary)
- Unripe fruit
- Acidic
- Fermented
- Remains strong with age

<u>Spicy</u>
- Peppers
- Activates the tongue by touch

Starchy (primary)
- *Carboplunk*-rich
- Digested like sugar
- Flour products (anything pulverized into a powder), breads, potatoes

Sweet (primary)
- Increases insulin energy
- Breast milk
- Fruit

This is all part of the science involved in preparing desirable food. Much research has been done in this area. It is worth learning the basics so you have more choices, adaptability and flexibility without sacrificing taste or health. My grandmother and my aunt were excellent cooks. They could walk into any kitchen with any amount of food and make a meal. I set a goal to be as capable as they were. When I learned about the science behind taste, preparing tasty nutrition became easier and more fun.

Being aware is fundamental to understanding the world we live in. It only takes a bit of education and learning a few skills to meet your nutrition needs. After that, it becomes pretty simple. There is no need to complicate nourishment and preparation with many ingredients and tons of spices. However, these types of recipes *can* be pretty amazing. The trick is getting real with your life and yourself.

I have conducted over 600 hypnotherapy sessions. Many have been past life regressions where the client visits and shares what is happening. This is a natural ability for most everyone. My job is to safely guide and ask questions that help the situation. In my weight loss sessions, I take people to a healthy life and to a point of time where they are sitting down to a family meal. Here, they are likely to be near a mirror to see themselves and to describe what is on the table.

Rome and ancient England are frequent healthy places they visit. They have much in common: meat, vegetables, fruit, water and/or wine. Through observance, there are no heavy sauces, *carboplunks*, deserts, grains, nuts or even bread. Grains, nuts, beans, ground flour and such may have been used, but they don't appear as relevant as the simple meat, fruit and vegetables that keep coming up in the sessions.

Everyone must eat to live. There is no reason to exchange

health for flavor. For example, dressings are incredibly simple to make if you understand a little of the science behind how the tongue and brain understand taste. It makes it easy to come up with all sorts of easy and correct combinations. A dressing can contain something sour (lemon juice), salty, savory (garlic), and a healthy oil. Whisk well, and you have a tasty dressing in the amount that you choose. With experience, you can mix something up that will eventually be a hit. There are so many ways a person can learn, and there are tons of highly rated recipes available.

Everyone tastes and responds to ingredients differently. Bud clusters can be in different areas on the tongue. Variations in cluster thickness can also affect flavor sensitivity. Our childhood food experiences can also heavily influence what is enjoyed or not. This can set the tone for being *carboplunk* tolerant.

India's Ayurvedic medicine considers the impact of free-flowing and blocked energy. This science is over 4,000 years old and is centered on three main parts to all living creatures. It is referred to as a science of life: *There is no mortality, only transformation.* This is a powerful viewpoint, and one I consider deeply. Cravings are heavily related to taste, healing and thinking.

Ayurvedic medicine relates cravings to specific organs, systems and healing needs. The healthy cravings are meant to sustain life; unhealthy cravings mask physical or energetic imbalances. Examples are craving food when the body needs water or craving fast foods and *carboplunks* for a pick-me-up when the body is looking for real nourishment. Unhealthy, non-nutritious cravings are confused brain communications. You taught the brain to think this way, so it supports you. The confusion is somewhere in the energy body (thought) and manifested through the physical body. This is why there can be physical and emotional withdrawals and resistance.

The body requires quality food with real nutrients, both energetically and physically. It is a form of awareness, respect and love to support the body in this way. Maybe your body loves and needs bitter tastes. Perhaps it's unable to eat a slice of fresh lemon because it is too strong and sour. The trick is being able to get past the influenced thinking so you can discover what the body truly wants. That requires getting rid of foods which get in the way of healthy choices. There will be adjustments. Give your tastes the needed time to heal from a *carboplunk* coma. Real food has flavors that are satisfying at every level.

It is unnatural to crave nutritionless foods with harmful ingredients like heavy metals, sawdust fillers, cancer causing and toxic ingredients, high sugar, unhealthy fats, etc. Nutrition must be a high priority. Give yourself a break.

Raising children with healthy nutrition habits is a lifelong gift. Children who eat well have a better chance of overcoming health challenges as adults. Unfortunately, many are raised on high sugar, high calories and *carboplunks*.

If you have ever known an adult who contracted Type 2 diabetes or had a gluten sensitivity, you've likely witnessed the result of excessive taste and cravings. The body demands a different way of eating. In these examples, there were tons of *carboplunks* involved. No one escapes their presence.

Much research has gone into finding ways to influence

our senses and the messages we get from them. Confusion is a key to addicting us to non-nourishing foods. Everything has positive and negative extremes; the senses are no exception. Businesses use every sense to aid in sales. Focus on what you can do, then do it. Balance, portions, variety and truth are the keys to maintaining a healthy nutritional approach. There is no reason to operate in fear, resistance and suspicion. You must be aware of the risks and tactics so you can protect, improve and maintain a quality of health emotionally and physically.

All of our senses come into play when it involves food; they can be our strength or our weakness. Allow the senses to be fed so the nourishing experience becomes even more satisfying. Here is a brief list of incredible "foodie" senses:

Hearing.

Bubbles exploding, sizzles and pops, crackles, crunches and snaps all add to the experience of eating. Cognitive neuroscience has revolutionized the food and beverage industry. Sounds shape our perception of foods and our receptiveness to suggestions intended to sway personal choice. Music and words are used in subliminal messages that humans cannot hear. Angry music can be used to irritate people in stores which can influence them to grab "calming" sugar items. I have watched people happily enter a store, hand in hand, and within 20 feet they start bickering with each other. Using unconscious sound is just another use of science to influence people. Recall the sound of a cool beverage being poured over ice on a hot day—very alluring.

Music can evoke all sorts of emotions and feelings.

Lower frequencies are calming and relaxing. Eighty beats per minute is considered the most comfortable tempo, and a steady volume is conducive to focused thinking. When sound is used to cause defiance, resistance or anger, every cell in the body is affected. It also lowers and dampens the energy body, making it more vulnerable.

Subliminal spoken messages have been around for decades and continue to be used today. On rare occasions, I have heard the words, *You want it. You want it now!* being repeated over and over behind a commercial or cleverly hidden behind the loud pop of a soda can being opened. This works on us, so be aware and be smarter!

Remind yourself before entering any store that these tactics are being used. They influence emotions and thoughts in hopes that it leads to impulse buying. I highly doubt the vegetable department is using these types of messages to suggest people buy vegetables. Rise above and refuse to fall for this. Choose to override with healthy choices.

Intuition.

There are limits to what is seen, felt and heard. The science of intuition involves techniques that measure psychic ability. This sixth sense has the ability to accurately define energetic and spiritual communication. It can alert you to things beyond what the physical senses can pick up. Those who use this sense are found to make faster, more accurate and more confident decisions.[17] Disconnection from this source means that a person must rely only on the 10% matter of

17 SAGE Journals; Galang Lufityanto, Chris Donkin and Joel Pearson, "Measuring Intuition: Nonconscious Emotional Information Boosts Decision Accuracy and Confidence, April 6 2016, Volume 27, Issue 5, https://doi.org/10.1177/0956797616629403

the physical body, which is 70% water. The body reacts to this communication and its subtle vibrational shifts, cluing us into what is needed or not needed.

These energetic sciences have been around for thousands of years. Edgar Cayce was the only person allowed to practice as a medical doctor without a license in the United States. Through hypnosis, he also found treatments to heal his patients. Tapping into the energetic field knowledge has been very successful. Governments and belief systems have spent decades studying these abilities. Psychics have been used (and still are) for remote viewing by every government. Animals have this skill, and children under age 4 have open connections. Even those who dismiss and debunk such skills as fraud make use of them.

To some extent, most (if not all) of us have the ability to receive messages from the energetic field. We are 6th sensory human beings, not 5. Developing these skills can be specific to the individual unless general skills are applied. Like any skill, this must be learned and developed to build accuracy.

Sight.

We often judge through sight regarding safety and appeal. We can make a decision on food based on color alone. Much research has gone into the visual effects and influences of color. Sight is one of the least trusted senses. Fooling others is nothing new; what you see is not necessarily what you get.

Let's apply sight to a portion and consumption example. It takes around 15 minutes for the body to send a message to the brain that it has had enough food. The eyes are indispensable in controlling the amount eaten. Try this basic rule:

stop eating when you feel about 70% full. There is no reason to overeat. It's uncomfortable, makes a person sluggish, disrupts sleep, overloads the digestion and adds unnecessary calories. Stop when you have eaten enough! In general, 2 cups of leafy vegetables, a small piece of protein and a cup of fruits and vegetables is all most people need on a daily basis. Allow your sight to let you know when you've had enough.

There are proven vibrational effects on cells, tissues, organs and other systems that regulate the body's functions, development and growth. Each color has its own frequency. When using color, it must be balanced with other colors in the spectrum so as not to overload. Reds have higher vibrations and blues have lower ones. A blue light near an exit door can be balancing. There is an art to combining color and light. In short, for every six uses of one predominant color, a complementary one (opposite color on the color wheel) should be used.

Each food has its own vibrational color effect when viewed and consumed. This goes beyond physical nutrition. Many Eastern medicines have extensive history using color vibrations to aid healing and mood through their connection with the cosmos and nature. Western medicine has used blue frequencies combined with warm light to stimulate a baby's liver to process and purge bilirubin (a waste product formed by cells dying and rejuvenating) naturally and safely. Clothing color can aid in establishing and portraying a mood through vibration and frequency communication. A red painted bedroom can disrupt sleep, while cooler blues can aid in relaxation.

When consuming a certain color of food at the right

time, we can influence a positive and self-caring change. If you have low energy, consume a red apple. Look at the brilliance of the color and appreciate it. This apple becomes a part of you and this relationship is what gives life. Intend to use the color vibration for its purpose. Be aware of how others use color to influence your purchasing dollars. Just because something is bright and glossy does not mean it is healthy or tasty. Real food has flavor that is far more satisfying than chemical-ridden, genetically altered and fake foods. It is also fun and healthy to connect with food in this way. Appreciation is a key to living mindfully. Become aware of what is going on around you, what you are doing and how you are feeling in this lovely world. Everything is connected. The more gratefulness we have, the more miraculous life becomes. Grace is a valued, spiritually connecting component of human development. It's what makes humans so caring, compassionate and kind.

Below are a few notes on basic colors. Keep in mind that color can be perceived differently. It has individual vibration and visual impact. No one views color exactly the same. All color is light. Without light there is no color. If a person reacts negatively to a color, their body is communicating that healing is needed. Scientifically, the focus is on vibration and wavelengths. Consider this generalized list when looking at and eating food.

Red (warm)

- Stimulating, exciting, passionate, action-oriented, draws attention, shows success, increases appetite, can be irritating and overwhelming

- Fruits, meats, vegetables with bright red skins, tomatoes, peppers
- Activates the 5 basic senses (hearing, seeing, smell, taste and touch)
- May help with migraines
- As lenses, can help with fall/winter seasonal affective disorder (SAD)
- Stimulates building red blood cells
- Complementary color is blue

Orange (warm)

- Decongesting, optimistic, rejuvenating, fun, friendly, bright, bold, cutting edge, good value, increases appetite
- Yams, oranges
- Healing
- Energizing
- A blend of red and yellow
- Complementary color is indigo

Yellow/Green (warm, neutral combination)

- Cleansing
- Green chili, lemons, limes
- Revitalizing, uplifting
- Cleansing foods

Green (neutral color, both warm and cool)

- Balancing, hopeful, growth, reassuring, refreshing, natural, organic, versatile, wealth, relaxing
- Fruits, dark leafy and other vegetables, olives, peas
- Master color in center of spectrum
- Good for skin
- No complementary color (opposite color that balances the energy); opposite is magenta

Turquoise (cool)

- Skin healing, calms the brain
- Aloe vera
- Fever and pain relief
- Combines green and blue
- Complementary color is lemon yellow

Blue (cool)

- Calming and soothing, detoxifier, trust, honesty, authority, serenity, intelligence, reliability, loyalty, reduces appetite
- Fish, veal, blue corn
- Fever and pain relief
- As lenses, can help with spring/summer seasonal affective disorder (SAD)
- Complementary color is red

Indigo (warm)

- Intuition, intelligence, tradition, seriousness
- Blueberries
- Fever and pain relief
- Spirit world connection
- Complementary color is orange

Violet (warm)

- Relaxes, calms lymphatic, anti-aging, princely
- Blue plums
- Fever and pain relief
- Controls hunger
- Destroys harmful bacteria
- Complementary color is yellow

Purple (neutral)

- Relaxes and calms emotions, creativity, spiritual, individual, quality, royalty, elegance, prestige, reduces appetite
- Blackberries, purple grapes
- Lowers blood pressure
- Relieves excessive pain from pressure
- Soothing for emotions
- Stimulates activity in veins
- Complementary color is scarlet

Magenta (neutral)

- Balance emotions, levels blood pressure, luxury, refined, rich
- Eggplant, beets
- Combines Red and Violet
- No complementary color; polarity is green

Yellow (warm)

- Uplifting, happy, enthusiastic, optimistic, friendly, confident, increases appetite, can be overwhelming and irritating
- Yellow apples, yellow corn
- Activates thymus gland (pain relief)
- Stimulates digestion

Scarlet (neutral)

- Speeds up heart rate, raises blood pressure, stimulates kidneys and adrenals
- Red cherries, strawberries
- Strongest of 12 healing colors
- Complementary color is purple

There are more possibilities and exceptions to this list. Love and respect color; it makes a difference in everything. How sad the world might be if there was only black and white.

Lastly, colors in the non-visible spectrum enter the eyes and aid in balancing hormones. Never stare directly at the sun, but being out in that radiant light does help with hormone balance.

Smell.

This totally works with and enhances taste. Scents are involved in behavioral science, neuroscience and advertising. They are picked up by the nose, which filters and helps the brain identify smells. The sense of smell can guide the body to nutrition or alert it to danger, such as with spoiled foods. Without smell, there is little ability to taste. There are 600,000 cells connected to the olfactory center. It is believed that the nose can detect over 1 trillion odors.[18] There is nothing like the smell of quality, real and flavorful eats.

Enjoy and use this sense with appreciation and gratefulness. It is most pleasurable and has no calories; it's a form of nutrition. Let the nose consume and incorporate a yummy scent as if it were food being consumed. This can also help a person eat less. Stores and restaurants use smell to entice. A cup of apple juice slowly simmering with cinnamon and nutmeg can be very bewitching. You can do the same at home. Smell something amazing, breathe it in and smile. Absorb it, enjoy it, breathe out and move on. It's a creative choice.

---

18 Scientific American, Jessica Morrison of Nature magazine, "Human Nose Can Detect 1 Trillion Odors," March 20 2014, https://www.scientificamerican.com/article/human-nose-can-detect-1-trillion-odors/

Sound.

As mentioned before, sound is very alluring. Chronobiology is the science of sound. It focuses on the fact that people should be in tune with their unique internal music. This a most beautiful thought because each person has her own vibrational song. People are instruments which are meant to be fine-tuned. We each have a different tone, rhythm and volume. When we are fine-tuned and connected with self and others, health and the Divine are at their highest.

External music affects heart rate, pulse, breathing, blood pressure, muscle tension, action, and has an electrical response from the skin. It can help increase endurance and muscle control and can also distract from something uncomfortable. It can improve an outlook and be entertaining and inspiring. Music speaks two universal languages: mathematics and geometry. Studies show that classical music aids in plant growth, while heavy, angry music kills them. Also, heavy and loud drumming can damage our brain cells and disrupt healthy vibrations in our body.

Music is medicine. It can be used for healing and to evoke deep forms of relaxation for strong and energetic spiritual connections. It can enhance or diminish learning, and so much more. If music is this powerful externally, imagine the potential for getting intensely connected with your own musical vibrations and qualities.

Music is a form of connecting with the atmosphere and with energy. The American natives have proven that song, when combined with focused thought and the actions of dance, can influence the atmosphere to cause rain or snow.

Imagine getting home from work. You're starving and just want to grab a *carboplunk*. Instead, you play some uplifting music while you enjoy a healthy salad in harmony. Immediately, you are singing and dancing around the kitchen, easily making healthy choices for vitality.

Texture.

Rheology is the science of food sensation in the mouth. It focuses on its consistency and flow. Psych rheology is an individual's view of a food's rheology. It's an entirely different science. For example, many believe a rougher texture is connected to sourness, so sugar is coated onto sour candy to compensate). Texture also alters your expectation about how you expect something to taste—the thicker the drink, the more creaminess is expected. Attitudes and perceptions play a huge role in how texture affects thinking about nutrition. No doubt these developed ideas originated externally from culture, family, belief system and regional indicators.

Texture increases aroma and increases taste by as much as 10 times.[19] Even though taste is similar, texture has a big influence. Without sight, smell and texture, it would be hard to tell what we are really eating. How a food feels affects its eating pleasure.

Chewing (mastication) is also part of texture. It is the first step to digestion. A baby moving from soft to more complex food can find it challenging because of the change in texture, not to mention chewing takes more effort. Chew-

19 Physiology & Behavior, Cees de Graaf, "Texture and satiation: The role of orosensory exposure time," May 15 2012, https://www.sciencedirect.com/science/article/abs/pii/S0031938412001953

ing increases saliva, which contains enzymes that help to break down the food. The better the chewing, the easier it is on the digestive system. As texture changes, that new information is sent to the brain. Texture during every step is also considered by manufactures and developers.

Take smaller bites. If you move your head forward like a turtle to help swallow a big clump of food, your bites are too big. Gulping food may be necessary from time to time, but you shouldn't make it a habit. It's much harder for the digestive system to break down large chunks, and nutrients can be missed because of it.

Thought.

This is linked to sensation, which is emotional. How a person thinks about what is consumed is huge. Many people think it is a treat to pile fast foods into their system, but it causes much emotional and physical damage. Fake food is cheap for a reason. A person will not get nutritional satisfaction from this. Instead, they will get a lower heart rate (from higher fat), increased bloating (from higher salt/sodium) and weight gain (from higher calories). There are also high levels of antibiotics, hormones, chemicals, fillers and sugar. Fast food is designed to be profitable and addictive. To me, this type of food is poison to the body.

When you prepare your own meals, that connection affects the energy of every item. Being mindful when preparing means you are appreciative and present in what you are doing. It connects with gratitude.

Genetically altered and cloned foods lack nourishment. Some farms and ranches raise their stock inhumanely. When an animal is in fear, adrenaline is raised and damages its meat. How we think affects every cell in our body. Animals and plants are no different. Fear is simply destructive. It is believed that under such stress, food has less physical nutrition and higher calories. This eventually undermines health.

It may help to think of it another way. When a person feels secure and loved, their senses are heightened and alive because love is an energetic nutrient! Food from nature is the same. It gave up its life or part of itself to support your life. It is certainly food for thought.

Touch.

External, internal, energetic and physical sensations are transmitted by the surfaces of foods and by reactions throughout the digestion processes. Haptic science is the communication and sensation of touch. Externally, it involves texture felt by the hands or other parts of the body. Internally, chewing is felt by the teeth and tissues of the mouth, throat and esophagus.

Sensations can reveal things the body no longer wants, such as spicy foods that cause acid reflux. Remove those items and the body calms down. It simply means the body no longer wants them. Popping an antacid is likely to make acid levels too low, so the body will react by creating more. Simply don't eat what the body doesn't like. When you listen and take action, the body will speak up clearer each time. Once in a while, popping a pill can be fine; but if this is consistent, other issues may be present. This is where outside guidance can be most beneficial.

Vibration and energy sense.

Energy senses include vision (light), hearing (sound waves) and touch (pressure); but they don't include the type of vibrational nourishment.

Everything in the Universe is based on vibrations and frequencies, and our nutrition is no different. Frequency and vibration have strong and subtle energies. Common sense tells us nourishment must contain live energy. Vibration can be measured in hertz. Here is a brief breakdown:

Food vibrations.

Fresh Foods: 20-27 Hz

Dried Foods: 15-22 Hz

Fresh Herbs: 15-22 Hz

Processed or Canned Foods: 0 Hz

Lower frequency attracts and absorbs negative energy like a sponge. When you are disconnected, altering yourself with drugs and alcohol or consuming unhealthy and low vibrational foods, the body and brain act and react at lower vibrations. These causes a person to be vulnerable and will likely attach to negative energy. Stress lowers vibration and makes the immune system vulnerable, allowing the body to be susceptible to diseases.

Nikola Tesla was a pioneer in electrical technology. He believed that if we avoid frequencies which interfere with the body, we can have greater resistance toward disease. According to Bruce Tainio (Tainio Technology), the average frequency of the human body is 62-68 Hz. A healthy body resonates between 62-72 HZ. Disease creeps in at 58 MHz, and our susceptibility to cancer begins at 42 MHz. Higher frequencies cause energetic changes in the body, lower frequencies make physical changes and middle frequencies affect emotional changes. The spiritual frequency range is between 92-360 Hz. It makes sense to consume nutrition higher in vibration.

Zingy mouthwatering taste.

I have no intention of leaving this earth feeling deprived of joy in eating tasty items. Taste buds are physical; they do not exist in energetic form. You cannot taste without taste buds. Allow yourself some taste pleasure. Learn how to create high quality, healthy and tasty dishes.

There is no good reason to ignore the basics. If there is no time to cook, eat simply by consuming items directly from the earth such as salads, fresh fruits and vegetables.

Think about good nutrition for the body. Refuse to spend dollars on items that do not serve your health. Unfortunately, there will always be long lines at the fast-food places. Many people don't care about their own health until they lose it. Make a better choice before that happens.

Be respectful of your precious body. It is such a gift to have so many varieties of healthy, organic and Kosher items from which to choose.

Changing how you think about nutrition and your body brings awareness that is both positive and respectful. Hopefully, you will be able to make smarter choices. Don't deprive yourself of flavor and wonderful taste. Let go of any excuse and find a balance between taste, nutrition and life.

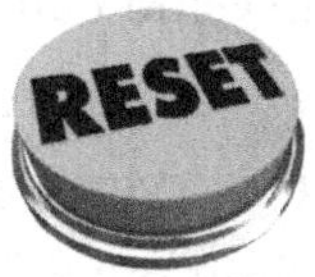

6| The Nitty Gritty on Nutrition

It is good sense and beneficial to have presence with nutritional items. Although the body is a bit different for everyone, there are similarities that can aid us in better health.

Diets.

Diet means the kinds of food a person eats. People eat what is locally available. In Australia, it is not uncommon to eat kangaroo. In Europe, fowl is highly common. Every landmass generally provides the local common food. Insects may sound horrible to you, but in Uganda they are a delicacy which provides tasty protein and nutrition. In Asian culture, fish eyes are a delicacy. Bisque and soups are common among all cultures.

Eating locally has its merits. Don't waste money on fad ideas. For example, obtaining a fruit from around the world with supposed healing properties might have been found locally. Of course, more remote areas with harsher environments may need to rely on foods from elsewhere in order to have a healthy variety.

Some foods have been associated with spiritual meanings; they've been included in ceremony, worshipped and connected to special events. When traveling, find out what is common around you. We can't expect others to have the exact items as our country and cultures. They all have their myths, fables, stories and commercialization around what they think is necessary to survive. When we step out of our comfort zones and dive into other living and eating experiences, we can learn so much.

Cultures can get so fixated in an idea that they ignore any science that could reveal harmful ingredients in their cuisine. This can make it hard to accept change. Furthermore, commercialization (by mega-corporations) continually pushes profitable items to other cultures. Countries with healthier diets that incorporate American *carboplunks* continue to have deteriorating health. It is a pharmaceutical and mega-corporation dream come true. It is up to you to see beyond this and rise above. Let go of any anger or complaining; this has been around for a long time. America has taken advantage of setting rules that support profit over health.

In some societies, it's a common approach in schools to teach children to grow organic vegetable gardens and to cook from scratch. The push for corporate profit is causing children to get further away from this. It is risky to let others determine what you put in your mouth. Everything you put into your mouth and on your body is medicine. It will either help or hurt.

It is beneficial to study other approaches. A common similarity around the world supports the concept of the body needing to be more alkaline than acid. Ancient Ayurvedic science has a detailed dietary approach. It includes balancing and harmonizing a person's energy, and it's based on a more alkaline diet. Qi gong is an amazing health approach that also involves the body, mind and energy. In similar healthy approaches, there are differences to be considered. In Ayurveda, onions are believed to heat the body and should be avoided; but in Chinese (Qi gong) nutrition, onions are considered to be a detoxifier and good for the body. Both approaches are thousands of years old. No one approach has all the answers, but it's definitely worth considering, especially if science is backing it up.

In America, alkaline diets are now being embraced. The Keto diet is an example; however, many diets, even this one, include *carboplunks*. Preprocessed and flour-type products are acidic. Get rid of the *carboplunks* to become healthier. Scientific approaches do change over time as we learn more. Keeping it simple is consistently easier and is supported by the different approaches.

Eating too much causes weight gain, stresses the digestive system, stretches out the stomach and causes much damage. It can feel awful. Nutrition from the earth (not canned, jarred or processed) is the best choice.

Did you know that peanut butter is allowed so many rat hairs per jar, or that jarred parmesan cheese and tea leaves in bags can contain a certain percentage of sawdust? These fillers are a waste of money and fill the tummy and body with unnatural items. If it is not nutritious for the body, then don't eat it. If you do, limit it. Limiting does not mean once a week; it means once in a great while or every few months. Better yet, avoid it as much as possible. Put your money where it gives the best health bang for the buck. These smart choices can ultimately affect company profits, so change may actually occur for the better.

Avoid excessive acid and acid-forming items in your diet. Make sure you consistently get plenty of alkaline items such as vegetables. As science has proven, sugary and salty items should be kept to a minimum. Even with healthier choices, consistently eating too much will likely cause more damage. Nutrition and variety are the most influential keys. If it is not nutritious for the body, don't eat it; but limit your portions if you do. Once a week is not limiting. Once every few months or longer is more like it.

The body needs to be surprised. It gets lazy with the same old routine. Sometimes I eat one meal a day, and sometimes I spread a meal throughout the day. I let my body tell me what it needs, but also try not to consume more than one meal in a day. My body does not need more. There is no one-size-fits-all solution, and no magic pill or surgery will ever work over time. You must make it an ongoing lifestyle.

Be truthful.

Some people change their eating styles before getting a blood test in the hopes of showing low cholesterol. Some of them dump excess weight before a medical appointment to show lower numbers on the scales. Doctors may think you are eating and living healthfully, but these efforts to manipulate tests are corrupt. These people will pay the price in the long run. Doctors are aware of these and other tactics, and it's not hard for them to determine the real story. People need to see and hear the truth. You cannot create change if it's based in foolery. Doctors have many patients, and they may not care either way how you choose. But your body will.

Medical professionals have many limitations, especially in Western medicine. They often tell their patients what they want to hear to avoid upsetting them. A client of mine was once told she had developed adult diabetes and that it was genetic. She was told she could have desserts as long as she ate a big salad to slow the digestion. Medical professionals know this is not true, but they also know patients will eventually figure it out. People are likely to make changes only when given enough of a reason to do so. Sugar is poisonous to the body, especially for those with diabetes.

My client ended up in the hospital after eating her dessert with salad. Only then was she willing to make changes—not before. Like many people, she had to experience the risk. Her focus changed to her health and lifestyle rather than being angry at the doctor.

It is easy to forget how trapped the medical community is. They must appease the patient, the hospital administrators, the Food and Drug Administration, insurance companies, the American Medical Association, the pharmaceutical industry and more. Complaints affect the doctor, the clinic and the hospital, which can lead to doctors being sued, getting fired or having their license pulled. They also may write your story down a bit differently than stated to avoid litigation situations. These are time-consuming, take them away from helping patients, and risky to their profession.

Doctors used to be the ones who decided what was best for their patients. Those days are gone. Today, they walk a very fine line so as not to upset or displease anyone. Telling a patient to be responsible and make better changes is a risk many may not be willing to take.

I have been approached by therapists, lawyers and a politician who have all attempted to get me to reveal something that could expose me to a lawsuit or shut down my business. There are regulations professionals must follow or risk being put out of business. There are far too many lawyers and individuals who look for easy targets as a way to make money and eliminate the perceived competition. It's sad and unfortunate that professionals must constantly be aware of this threat.

Diabetes and genetics.

With diabetes, insulin (necessary to break down sugar) stays at high levels over time. Because these levels are always high, the body stops recognizing it and doesn't regulate it. Now insulin must be regulated by medicine. Adult diabetes (type 2) in some is reversable, but it must involve a full lifestyle change in how, when and what people eat and drink. Even if people are genetically predisposed, they are not powerless.

Too often, genetics are blamed for diseases. This can deter people from making otherwise healthy lifestyle changes. If obesity runs in the family, stop eating the way they do. If heart disease is prevalent, don't be as idle as they are. You may need to be more determined and attentive to avoid genetic sensitivity, but it doesn't necessarily mean you are doomed. You have a choice.

Around the world, studies have shown that you can override genetics. Genetic sensitivity can be lessened by the actions and nutrition you choose. Because illness and disease are profitable, it can be difficult to manage this within the medical industry. Rise above all the influences and do things differently.

The physical body speaks up in so many ways that are unique to the individual. The darker aspects of the world try to convince us there is little choice. They specifically target how you think and feel about each other, the world, your Creator, the Universe and ourselves. We must help each other find ways to rise above it all to become the healthy beings we are meant to be.

With so much information and knowledge being shared these days, we are all very connected in spite of those who wish to undermine our efforts. Everything we see and hear can be altered to spread misinformation that supports hidden agendas. Share with others and overcome sabotaging beliefs and thoughts. This is a journey of discovery that continues throughout life. There is strength in numbers and like-mindedness. As our mental, physical and spiritual health all rise, so will the power of truth and positivity.

Do not rely on anyone to decide for you. It is an honor and a privilege to make your own decisions. Determining truth is a skill. As you read literature, feel the sensations and emotions that rise within and around your body. Notice your attitudes and the thinking behind them. Discover what works for you.

Relax, get tuned into the soul, and pay attention to first reactions and thoughts that occur. Determine truth for yourself and do not make it complicated. Be honest with yourself and refuse to become overwhelmed. Take it one step at a time and one change at a time, then see the difference it makes. Always move forward.

The body speaks.

This is an individual exploration. The physical body speaks up in so many ways that are similar and unique to each other and the individual. The following list shows a few conditions worth paying attention to. Most can be avoided with proper hygiene. Make note of what you ate, drank or are stressing about.

- Hard and/or loud forced belching: *swallowing air, oversized bites, carbonation, eating too fast, stress*
- Bad breath: *digestive issues, poor hygiene, lungs, stomach, illness, stress, dehydration*
- Body odor: *food eaten, stress, overconsumption of alcohol/drugs, low in minerals or vitamins such as zinc, toxins, imbalanced hormones*
- Acid reflux: *not enough stomach acid, wrong foods, too spicy, too many carboplunks, blood pressure, stress*
- Smelly gas: *wrong foods, dehydration, stress*
- Highly smelly poop: *too many carboplunks, health imbalance, stress*
- Constipation: *dehydration, wrong foods*
- Smelly or cloudy urine: *types of food and beverages consumed, kidney complaints, bacteria*
- Stomach ache: *eating too fast, wrong foods, stress*
- Digestive pain: *wrong foods, eating too fast, not chewing well, intestinal issues, dehydration, stress*
- Weight gain: *too much food, wrong foods, stress, eating at wrong times, health issues*
- Quick weight loss: *health issues, stress, imbalances*
- Dry mouth: *dehydration, stress, digestive issues*

- Dry skin: *dehydration, health issues, not enough healthy oils, stress, climate*
- Rash on skin: *stress and many other possibilities*
- Sores on skin: *stress and many other possibilities*
- Hiccups: *dehydration, stress, eating too fast, wrong foods*
- Twitching: *stress, neurological or neuroemotional issues*
- Diarrhea: *too many toxins, wrong foods, stress*
- Dry scalp: *dehydration, climate adjustments, other issues*
- Constant runny nose: *dehydration, illness*
- Frequent illness: *immune issues, lack of cleanliness*
- High LDL cholesterol: *wrong foods, liver complaints*
- Sluggishness: *wrong foods, stress, sleep issues, emotional issues*
- Foggy head: *gluten or other food sensitivity, sleep issues, emotional issues, stress*
- Headaches: *dehydration, sleep issues, gluten or other food sensitivities, stress*
- Nausea: *diabetes, wrong foods, eating too much, stress, illness, infection*
- Vomiting: *illness, infection, stress, diabetes, wrong foods, food sensitivity*
- Mucus in the throat, lungs or poop: *food sensitivity, wrong foods or beverages, dehydration*
- Itchy skin: *not enough healthy oils, dehydration, stress*
- Dry eyes, floaters in the eye, cataracts: *dehydration, lack of healthy oils, stress, environment, eye issues*

- Excessive bloating: *wrong foods, dehydration, not chewing properly, stress*
- Inflammation: *wrong foods, dehydration, too much salt, injuries, lack of exercise, stress*
- Highly smelly sweat (healthy sweat smells sweet): *wrong foods and beverages, dehydration, addiction or excess issues, stress*
- Racing heart: *too much caffeine, too much sugar, sensitivity, dehydration, lack of exercise, stress*
- Urgency to pee: *bacteria, kidney issue, dehydration*

If any of these are occurring and are *not* due to what is consumed, look at the things you are stressing about and find a different way to cope. Check with your doctor.

Diagnostics.

Make certain that proper diagnostics are being done. Guessing is common in the medical industry because similar symptoms can present across several diseases and illnesses. Without a diagnostic confirmation, it's usually just a good guess. Choose wisely and reasonably. Diagnostics are costly, and it's common for the medical community to avoid these additional costs.

About 30% of people who get chemotherapy do NOT have cancer! I read this from a journal many years ago, but it seems there are controls in place. This study has been removed, even from the archives. Western doctors are not allowed to recommend alternative forms of therapy that have proven to be successful. All cultures have had to deal with cancer in the past and present. All have had their failures and successes.

I have had a naturally high red blood cell count since 2008. I used an alternative therapy in my 20s (Don Quai herb) which raised the cell count; it has never gone down. It's rare that red blood cells don't return to normal amounts. Stress was a serious issue. Due to the high red blood cell count, the oncologist had a JAK2 marker test done. This can aid in the identification of a specific cancer. The test showed a high indication. Doctors wanted to do immediate aggressive chemotherapy. I refused because the body can show symptoms before a person actually comes down with something. I asked for a bone marrow biopsy (very painful), which shockingly showed I did not have the rare cancer yet! I changed my life and my thinking to drastically lower stress. That lowered the marker, and it has remained low to this day.

My life was a huge struggle, but I embraced it and continued to take steps to improve my life. I discovered how a person can change one's thinking immediately. Thinking is designed to be flexible and adaptable, not rigid and limited. For example, you enter a job interview with a different mindset than entering a classroom. If you feel any level of defensiveness or negative emotion, stop. That thinking is not working, so change it to the positive. The easiest way to change thinking is to clear the mind, listen, look for opportunities to ask questions, observe with the intent to learn, and smile.

When I tore my rotator cuff in five places, I had to go through a year of insurance-required physical therapy, then had a proper diagnosis and surgery. The muscle could not heal without the tears being closed. Never skip physical therapy after any invasive or disruptive injury. It aids the body in regaining lost strength and range of motion, and those professionals have outstanding knowledge.

Learn to read your body, listen to it, get professional advice and take action. Naturally healing and keeping a body and mind healthy takes time, persistence and much patience. Pills, teas, herbs or specific foods alone will not heal, but they can aid the body in maintaining while the mind is healed first. A healthy mind is more apt to develop healthy cells. These are not long-term fixes, but choosing natural and alternative ways is certainly a better choice when appropriate. In some cases, medicine and symptom relief are absolutely necessary. The physical body does have limitations and may need extreme help at times. All approaches have their value.

Vibrational healing.

All life is vibration and frequency. There has been a recent breakthrough with vibrational relief in the treatment of Parkinson's disease. Kinesiology is a means of muscle testing that helps determine what the body is trying to say. It's a good check point for accuracy when done by a properly trained professional. The trick is to find the combination that works for you. Regardless of your choice, the most healing vibration is from thinking. Our brain and body are powerful healing instruments.

Sharing and overcoming sabotaging beliefs and thoughts is healing. It's a journey of discovery that continues throughout life. Embrace solving problems in this area and in life. There is strength in numbers and in like-mindedness. As the mental, physical and spiritual health of individuals rise, the power of truth and positivity also increases.

Any holistic wellness consultation should consist of:

- Improving the immune system, energy levels, hormonal balance and cognitive health.
- Digestive health
- Sleep quality
- Reducing stress
- Lessening inflammation
- Education in holistic health, alternatives, positive life changes and how to improve health
- Getting a strategic plan designed to improve health and well-being
- Getting to a root cause
- Sharing how changes will affect the relationship with yourself, environment, work and others
- Quality professionals asking questions of their clients

My clients have benefited from all of these. They have received a list of books to change or broaden thinking, techniques to help in specific health goals, a 12-page Nutritional Guidance packet (now part of this book), and better health and self-awareness concepts (emotionally and physically). It's enough to give them one to two years of individual work. There is no need for numerous appointments unless they want other services or wish to continue their healing journey at deeper levels. Healed clients give quality alternative professionals the most satisfaction and pleasure.

Alternative professionals believe in what they do, are passionate, professional and live what they believe. It is a mind, body and spiritual approach to living. Professionals do not bad mouth others and should embrace the positive side of all approaches, even Western.

What works for some may or may not work for you. This is where common sense and listening to that inner voice which recognizes truth come into play. Spirit leads and urges us toward healing, but it can be difficult to determine what we need specific to our health, which is why guidance from within is so important. The alternative field does have charlatans and fakes who harm its reputation with improper education or skills. No industry is immune to these. Check credentials (including medicinal approaches) and their willingness to refer a client to others who are qualified. Quality professionals admit their limitations.

If regulations govern what the alternative professional is practicing, make sure they are approved. Some states have higher requirements and others have little to none. Do your homework and don't waste time with anyone you feel uncomfortable with.

Reputation and word of mouth are highly important. It only takes one client to ruin a person's ratings, even if that person is highly skilled and successful in his/her field. If you feel calm around a professional or feel comfortably drawn in when he/she speaks, you are sensing truth and expertise. Professionals may speak kindly, but must also speak the truth. They should also ask clarifying questions to ensure they are on the right path with your specific needs. If not, then reconsider!

Do not stand for fluffy, indirect answers or the silent treatment. These are common in many Western industries, including medicine, dental, veterinary, mechanical and food.

Your questions should be answered; if not, the professional should ask further questions to better understand what you are seeking.

Embrace the power of choice.

It is an honor and a privilege to make your own decisions. The world often banks on you wanting to give up and allow someone else to decide for you. Rarely does this work in your favor. Learn to ask questions and require real answers.

Check your attitudes. Many of my clients and friends thought they didn't need to worry about their weight after they turned 60. Appropriate weight, specific to each body, brings vitality. People quickly realize how uncomfortable and damaging obesity can be to their lives and attitudes. People often live for another 30-50 years. Living with inappropriate weight can take over a person's livelihood and wallet. It's not worth it.

Determining truth and getting in touch with the power within you is a skill that is earned. When you read, feel the sensations and emotions that rise within and around your body. Notice the attitudes and thinking behind them. These are clues; it's like being a personal detective. Make it fun and don't beat yourself up. This is a journey in self and healing education. Stay open-minded and find what works for you.

As a person searches for the right approaches, the law of attraction sends both good and bad. You are meant to learn and get in touch with this super-power within. Sometimes, being wrong can lead to growth and is intended to happen, which is why it must always be considered as a possibility whether it's the professional or the client/patient. Each time you find a helpful approach, it will often lead you to the next step. Don't give up! Solving problems is what life is about.

Relax, get tuned into the soul and pay attention to your first reactions and thoughts. Determine truth for yourself and do not make it complicated. Keep it simple, be honest with yourself and refuse to become overwhelmed. Take it one step at a time, one change at a time, and see the difference it makes. Then move forward.

Whether you want a quick-fix solution or a long-term one, it's still your choice. Never push your decisions on anyone else. This is a stay-in-your-lane thing. What you choose may be absolutely right for you but totally wrong for another.

Important Mentions and Expanded Repeats

Body dampening.

Body dampening is a Chinese medicine term which means that a person's body is going through heavy stress. It can be caused by an accident, a close family death, a healing crisis, or anything that puts the body over the top. In body dampening, the digestive system gets so stressed out trying to digest that it depletes energy from the body. It's similar to a hot flash, but may not be as strong. If you feel your body heating up during or after eating, take action to alleviate the stress in life and with the body.

Lightly cook most all vegetables and fruits, add quality broths or soups, and do what you can to make it easier on digestion. Take time to relax after eating or go for a calm and gentle walk, as long as it does not heat the body. It's easy to overlook how life's stresses can affect the body.

Even if you don't experience body dampening, you know when things are getting hard on the body. Moving can be very stressful; so can a new job or anything that challenges your health. In these situations, consider treating the body as if it were dampened and give it some relaxation as mentioned above. The body is your universe. Take actions to keep it balanced before it needs to tell you something is wrong. There will always be times of imbalance. You cannot rebalance at a different level without it. Seeking constant balance can undermine growth. Both have their place in our experience and evolution here. Avoid harsh judgments of others and self. This only stagnates and blocks the opportunities that imbalance supersedes.

Breathing.

You are meant to use the lower abdomen when breathing. This is how babies breathe naturally. Our breathing eventually becomes shallow because many believe it makes us look fatter when we relax the lower abdomen. Shallow breathing is not healthy; it allows the buildup of toxins in the lower lungs. The Shaolin Kung Fu martial art teaches us to release all the air in the lungs to purge this buildup. Exhale, forcing out the air until none remains; then inhale. Be careful not to hyperventilate or pass out. Three cycles in a row is sufficient.

When breathing correctly, the lower abdomen fills up and the chest rises. Watch how a baby breathes; they do this. The reverse occurs when breathing out. If people think this makes a person look fat, then too bad! Your health is more important than the opinions of others. Do the best you can with what you have and what you can afford to work with. If you're uncomfortable breathing this way around others, do it when alone every chance you can.

Rhythmic breathing is a way to lessen pain and calm down. Breathe in and hold for a moment, then breathe out and hold for a moment. Repeat three times. This biologically calms the physical body and is a great way to relieve stress.

Sleep.

During sleep, the body repairs itself. There are a multitude of things that can affect a person's consistent rest such as nutrition, hydration, electromagnetism, light, colors, illness, disease, hormones, sounds, medications, muscle relaxation, tension and stress. Keeping a journal can be most effective in determining what patterns in life could be affecting your sleep.

Avoid eating 3-1/2 hours before bedtime, and avoid exercise 4 hours before bedtime. Studies have shown that people sleep better in dark rooms with no light. Try covering small lights to help darken the room. In the morning, allow sunlight to hit your face for about 15 minutes. Don't stare at the sun, but let its light touch your eyes. Sunlight contains the full spectrum of colors (visible and invisible) which enter the iris and aid in balancing hormones. It also helps to reset our biological clocks (circadian rhythm), which regulate wakefulness and sleepiness. Blue light from electronics and television screens have been found to disrupt sleep.

Add full-spectrum lighting everywhere you can. It can help you feel more energetic during the day and sleep better at night. Sleeping in a cooler environment is better than warmer. Also, using a light therapy device as an alarm is a more natural way to awaken. Gong alarms begin slowly, then increase, which is also natural. Remove all electrical impulse devices from the body, like watches. These affect our natural biological clocks.

It is advised that people eat a protein dense breakfast because breakfast (4-5 almonds is all you need if breakfast is not normally your choice) and morning exercise affect the circadian rhythms, the body's natural internal clock that directly affects sleep and waking. Proper circadian rhythms promote consistent restorative sleep and overall mental and physical health. *Carboplunks* and protein are not good companions. Protein with vegetables is helpful for proper digestion of the protein due to the vegetables containing and promoting the necessary digestive enzymes. Sleeping in a cooler environment is better than warmer. Using a light therapy device as an alarm is a more natural way to awaken. Gong alarms that start slowly before increasing can also be helpful. Remove all electrical impulse devices (watches, etc.) from and near the body. These also affect the natural biological clock.

Consider eating an apple 20 minutes before bedtime to raise blood sugar so it can then fall to promote more sleepiness. Medications at bedtime can cause a person to not get the required amount of deep sleep. If you must do this, limit them to three days in a row (maximum) to avoid psychological dependency. Troubled sleep can be an indication that something in life or health is out of balance.

Eliminate sugar, caffeine and gluten to see if any of these are affecting rest. Irritating and toxic relationships and stresses from work or home can affect sleep. Hydration is also important for sleep. Rule out (with a professional) other causes like thyroid, sleep apnea or hypertension.

There are great sleep music and sleep sounds available. This music is designed to work with brain waves, guiding them into relaxation and deep sleep. I find those designed at 432 Hz are the most effective.

The body responds to visualization and words. Picture a gorgeous setting that is cozy and comfortable. Say things to yourself such as *I love to sleep. I love to be comfortable in my bed and on my pillow. It feels so wonderful to rest.* Keep these positive and do not let yourself go negative.

Set a routine before bedtime; it's an effective approach. It prepares the brain and body for what is about to happen.

If a person is not dreaming, this too can be an indication of a lack of life awareness and/or spiritual development. Dreams are meant to release frustrations, fears, confusion and stress. Many times, problems can be solved while sleeping. They can be a form of energetic communication to aid and guide you. Paying attention to dreams, especially between 2:00-4:00 am, can be profound.

Thyroid.

This a very important gland for weight management. Consider having this checked to see if it is underactive or overactive. If the condition is minor, it can easily be modulated with diet and exercise.

Foods that are high in sulfur and/or contain goitrogens can interfere with iodine and other minerals necessary for a healthy thyroid. There are three types of goitrogens: goitrins, thiocyanates and flavonoids.

Goitrins and/or thiocyanates.

> bamboo shoots, babassu (coconut fruit in Brazil and Africa), bok choy, broccoli, Brussels sprouts, cabbage, cassava root (African), cabbage, canola, collards, corn, cauliflower, daikon, flax, kale, kohl-rabi, lima beans, linseed, millet, mustard, peaches, peanuts, pears, pine nuts, radishes (including horse-radish), rapeseed (canola oil), rutabagas, spinach, strawberries, swedes, sweet potatoes, turnips and watercress are some of the foods that contain these ingredients.

Lightly cooking any of the above will help shut down and break down the goitrogen so it is no longer an issue. Balance these out with rich iodine (kelp, kombu, nori, wakame seaweeds, cod, shrimp, tuna, eggs, prunes) and selenium (Brazil nuts, fish, meat, sunflower seeds, baked beans, portobello mushrooms, whole grain pasta, cheese) foods.

Unfortunately, the following foods also contain goitrogens for which heating will not shut them down:

> soy and soy-based foods such as edamame, soy milk, tofu, tempeh

I eat very little soy and make sure to get plenty of iodine and selenium-rich foods to balance it out. Soy also can affect the proper absorption of thyroid-balancing hormones.

Flavonoids.

These are found in bark, berries, grains, red wine, roots, stems, flowers and teas. Flavonoids can cause nausea, headache and tingling in the arms, hands or feet. Tea can actually be associated with liver toxicity and are often dehydrating. However, they can be helpful to your health when used correctly.

When thyroid functions are disrupted, important hormones that regulate metabolism are affected. This can lead to issues with body temperature, heart rate, protein production, calcium, and how the body deals with fats and carbohydrates (healthy and unhealthy).

Consume small amounts of these and take precautions. Cook those that can be, and balance them out with other foods (like lots of vegetables) to balance out a little soy. Those above also contain health benefits. Have a variety and mix it up.

Necessary Awareness and Considerations (these guidelines are flexible)

Beans.

As with most things, these can be controversial. Beans contain phytochemicals (shown to lower heart disease) and cancer reducing chemicals such as isoflavones and phytosterols. They also contain high fiber and steady the glucose levels. Beans are also high in protein, vitamin E, B and much more. However, beans, grains and nuts contain phytic acid which binds to nutrients in foods and prevents you from absorbing them.

The lectins in beans can cause digestive problems such as nausea, vomiting, stomach irritation and even diarrhea. Lectin also may block the absorption of iron, phosphorus, zinc and calcium. Lectins are lessened, but not removed, by slow cooking on low heat and replacing the water they are soaked. If sprouting beans, it is wise to remove the outer hull. Some outer hulls on beans and peas have been linked to gout. Those with serious illness such as multiple sclerosis or irritable bowel syndrome should avoid beans.

In many areas of the world, beans are a main part of the diet. Beans contain some protein, but only in comparison to breads and vegetables. They can quickly raise carbohydrates to a point above what the body needs. This can contribute to weight gain and metabolic issues like insulin resistance.

Chickpeas and pinto are my favorite, but I do not eat them often. Black beans have good protein and other nutrients; but in general, beans aren't very important and mostly just add more starch.

Brain.

The brain requires nutrition and LDL cholesterol to bring in healthy oils. The brain is mainly energy and fat. For every serving of bad fat in the diet, there must also be three good fats. This is a balance.

Everything you see and place into the mind is there forever. Negative content will give rise to negativity in thinking and in life. Refer to this book's section on PTSD. There are many kinds of trauma; most people have experienced at least one or more event in their lifetime.

The brain needs exercise or it will get lazy. It will wire itself to support your way of thinking. Use it or lose it! The brain is like a muscle that needs exercise. Any group or organization that believes their world view is absolute can be a tragedy to brain health.

Calories.

Calories count. How wonderful that so many restaurants include calorie information in their meals. It can be a big deterrent to see a 1,900-calorie meal compared to a 400-calorie item. Counting calories is tedious, so learn to eat just enough but not too much. This is where organic foods can be very helpful. An organic apple, for example, is higher in nutrients and lower in calories than a non-organic or genetically altered apple (which is often much larger). Learn to eat foods high in nutrients in appropriate sizes. Your eyes can help. If the apple is larger, eat half the apple and have the rest the next day. Incidentally, the brown color that forms on the inside of the apple is just from oxygen exposure. It's not really a big deal, but go ahead and cut it off if it is to you.

A quarter to a half cup of vegetables is a proper serving. Have two cups of leafy greens a day, a sliced-up tomato (acid), half an avocado and some protein. Protein contains enzymes that aid in the absorption of nutrients from vegetables. A few raw almonds and prunes (protein and potassium) are tasty and filling for a nice breakfast.

When making a smoothie, be sure you know the calories, as some can be very high. You do not have to drink a 600-calorie smoothie all at once. Drink half in the morning and half for lunch. Eating out is most always high calorie. There is no reason to finish a large meal. Eat half the meal, then have the remainder the next day. Order soup and/or a salad instead of an entrée. The idea is to be wise. If you are gaining weight, you're consuming too many calories. To lose weight, there must be fewer calories and/or more exercise. It's pretty straightforward.

The rule of thumb is to consume 10 times the desired weight in calories. For example, if your desired weight is 140 pounds, multiply that by 10 to get 1,400 calories a day. Of course, this also depends on your activity level and other factors such as muscle mass and height, but it's a general formula.

Canned foods.

These foods are highly processed and contain no real energetic nutrition. They often contain heavily added salt/sodium, sugar, corn products and other ingredients that give flavor and extend shelf life. These can be convenient and are okay as an added item on occasion, but should never be a staple in any home. Much nutrition is lost in the processing, and the quality of the contents can be questionable. Dehydrating can be a good alternative.

Carbohydrates.

There are crappy carbohydrates such as processed items, flour products and sugar. There are also quality carbohydrates like fresh fruits, brown rice (arsenic-purged), leafy greens and vegetables. Some bodies require more fruits; some do better with vegetables, more or less. For me, an apple or kiwi and a few prunes are enough, or maybe some blueberries and mango. To make up for nutrients, use a super dehydrated fruit and vegetable mix from time to time.

Fruits are best consumed by themselves and not mixed with other foods. Eat them two hours before anything else and 20-30 minutes after other foods. This is not always reasonable, but citrus is more flexible. Do what you are willing to. It's worth keeping in mind.

The more you rid yourself of crappy carbs, the less cravings you'll have. The body wants nutrition, not crap.

Cheese.

This is not a very digestible item. It clogs arteries and does not have enough nutrition to justify its consumption. It's a bit of calcium protein, phosphorus, B12 and A vitamins with little else. It is high in salt and creates a stringy digestive mess. Hard cheeses are easier on the stomach and contain less sugar. There are many contradicting articles on cheese, so it's hard to determine accuracy. Mozzarella, goat and Swiss are lower in sodium, and cottage cheese has lower calories which make these healthier choices. Avoid eating cheese on a consistent basis. Eat small amounts and take breaks from it. It's okay to indulge on occasion, but limit this food in your diet. It's mainly just a tummy-filler.

Cholesterol.

These are lipoproteins—HDL (healthy/good cholesterol) and LDL (lousy/bad cholesterol). Both are needed! The liver makes cholesterol. It is also found in some foods such as dairy and meat. LDL cholesterol is what carries needed fats to the brain. Without it, the brain does not get the nutrients it needs.

Cholesterol-lowering medication should be used with caution. Determine if the liver itself is responsible for higher levels (genetics) by correcting the diet for a couple of months and retesting to see if levels improve. Stop smoking, get rid of excess weight, consider any medications being taken or any diseases that may be present, then retest again. Too many people take this type of medication without first changing the diet to determine if the liver is responsible for over-producing. In taking cholesterol-lowering medication, though, people can be misled into thinking they can continue eating the same (or more) items which naturally raise LDL. This thinking is unhealthy. Less than 100 mg of LDL is considered optimal *(MedlinePlus.gov, U.S. National Library of Medicine: LDL: The "Bad" Cholesterol, also called: Low-density lipoprotein. Look under Home, Health Topics, LDL: The "Bad" Cholesterol).*

Cacao.

The best way is the natural way. Get these nuts separately, crush them up and add to a smoothie; or eat 2 or 3 to get the best benefits. When processed, cacao loses many of its benefits. Dark chocolate does not have the same benefits as the original fresh or dried nut. I grind the dried nuts in my coffee grinder and store in a tightly closed container in the refrigerator. Any excess nuts are also stored this way.

Coffee.

Everything in moderation is the rule. The body needs variety. Coffee is acidic, and its caffeine should be a consideration. There are many healthier alternatives with the same pick-me-up that coffee gives. Check out the honey and cinnamon drink in the *Tips and Tricks* chapter. Change things up to surprise the body and the taste buds. Adding sugar, milk or flavorings increases the calories and negates any benefit it might otherwise have. Coffee also stains the teeth, so give the mouth a break.

With all the fancy, sugar-filled coffee beverages at fast food places, this can be a difficult addiction when combining caffeine and other ingredients. Coffee is highly profitable, by the way. Health-wise, it's really not in a person's best interest.

If you are person who consumes coffee throughout the morning and day, you are setting yourself up for serious kidney issues down the road. In addition, a cup of coffee is NOT a mug of coffee. When you remove coffee for a while, notice if you get irritable and/or agitated. The body will scream for the addictive substance you have been giving it. Change things around and get less dependent on coffee.

As with any addiction, try to quit gradually over time. Don't quit right before an important event or something big. Begin the withdrawal during down times such as when you're ill or otherwise off your routine. It gets easier after the first week. Go ahead and have a cup for an occasional pick-me-up. As with any drug, take in moderation.

If you experience any sign of a kidney or bladder problem, or are healing something like bone, give up caffeine. It is hard on the organs, skeleton and digestive system.

Corn.

Corn is basically sugar to the body, and it has few nutrients. Most items made with ground corn are actually from feed corn. If a person is prone to gaining weight easily, see how much corn might be in his/her diet. It fattens people as easily as it fattens cows.

Sensitivity to corn is common. It is in many things such as malt, hamburger patties, taco meat, puddings, many beverages, yogurt, salad dressings, mayonnaise, soup mixes, beans, many baked goods, vanilla extract, baking powder, modified starches, gravy, peanut butter, Vitamin D fortified milk and many plastic bottles. It's also in vegetable oil; anything battered in this (fries, chicken, etc.) will absorb it. Animals fed corn will have as much as 42-50% in their meats and eggs. Many foods contain corn because it is cheaper than other products.

Dairy.

Processing destroys enzymes, which makes it more difficult to absorb nutrients. I can eat cheeses in limited amounts, and I use buttermilk (less calories than regular milk) in cooking on rare occasions. Otherwise, mucus forms in my throat immediately (the body speaks). I do not believe we are meant to be drinking milk after young childhood. No other animal consumes milk as it ages; the animals know better than we do.

If you must have dairy, use organic and avoid growth hormones, steroids, antibiotics and other chemicals found in animals' feed. This should not be consumed daily, but studies are highly conflicting. It must be an individual decision based on what the body is telling you.

Those who consume dairy have a higher rate of broken bones as they age. Yogurt has some health benefits. It's a milk product and is fine on occasion, but I do not believe daily consumption is healthy for most people. Again, it depends on the body.

There are some benefits to yogurt, but in limited amounts. Additives such as flavorings, oils, sugar and preservatives undermine any health benefit. Yogurt is a pasteurized item, so it loses nutrients in favor of a longer shelf life. Probiotics added to yogurt can be a problem when consistently consumed. These are made naturally from good bacteria and yeast. They help get rid of the bad. These are often recommended after antibiotic use because antibiotics kill off yeast and the good and bad bacteria. If you get diarrhea after use, you do not need them. Don't become dependent on these. Seek out probiotic balance naturally.

There is controversy over low-fat items about how the fat is removed and what is used to remove it. Historically, milk had a bit of an aftertaste, but now it no longer does. Nothing on the label mentions what might have been used to cover up the aftertaste.

If mucus builds up in the throat or lungs after consuming a dairy product, stop consuming it.

Carboplunks and protein do not mix. Cereal is a ground type of flour and nothing but a *carboplunk.* It raises blood sugar drastically, regardless of what any of the so-called studies say otherwise. Dairy is a huge industry. Weeding through the studies is extremely confusing and full of contradictions.

No client of mine during any past-life hypnosis session has ever mentioned milk or dairy in their environment. When people lived on farms and ranches, they consumed fresh milk and butter. It was much healthier, and hard work kept their calories and fat to a minimum.

I don't believe in fake butter. It often uses unhealthy oils to cut back on the calories. Limit its use and always choose unsalted and organic. Real butter from an organic ranch or farm is the best, but not very accessible to most.

Condiments.

These enhance many items, but often contain high salt/

sodium, sugar, colorings, unhealthy oils, flavorings and the like. Use them sparingly. Dressings are delicious and easy to make at home using less salt/sodium and sugar. A sandwich doesn't necessarily need an added condiment. Smothering potatoes in high-sugar ketchup depletes any nutritional value and only increases calories.

Find ways to limit or eliminate the use of so many condiments. Even mayonnaise, honey or sugar can be present in homemade dressings. A simple squeeze of a lemon with a little added garlic can be very tasty. Add some quality olive oil to take it to another level. Always control the amount; too much dressing can cause the oil to block the nutrition. A little goes a long way. Eating a salad without a dressing is just fine.

Enjoy a condiment on occasion. Find healthier alternatives such as using avocado instead of mayonnaise or maybe a little mustard; but watch these very closely.

Dehydrated foods.

Dehydrating foods is easy and they retain their energetic nutrition. It's a great way to plan ahead. Dehydrating green onions at their peak makes them available year-round. Dehydrating already frozen organic blueberries and mango chunks works great and is a good time-saver. I top my salads with the blueberries and carry some mango in my purse for a quick snack. A piece or two of dehydrated beef in the freezer is handy, as well. Dehydrators are helpful, but not necessary; the process is just as efficient in the oven. Keep in mind these foods can stick to the teeth and promote tooth decay. Always brush the teeth 20-30 minutes after eating. Many things can be dehydrated, including full meals and soup mixes.

Desserts.

Many years ago, I made a rule that I would not have desserts unless I made my own. Desserts are full of unhealthy fats, flour, sugar, salt, flavoring, preservatives, colorings and more. They can be addicting and cause cravings for foods with no health benefits. Don't fall for the cliché that it's not a real meal without dessert. There are many ways to make a dessert without unhealthy choices.

Try slicing an apple and add a small amount of butter, sugar, pure maple syrup, cinnamon and nutmeg. Cook it until soft. It's just as wonderful without a pie crust or topping. If you must have a dessert, avoid the prepared ones. This includes any high sugar items.

Eggs.

These are a great source of protein. If you are concerned about cholesterol and fat, you can remove most (not all) of the yolk. Try boiling them to avoid having to add fat. Store boiled eggs in the refrigerator. Place them in a covered bowl with a bit of water or a wet paper towel. This will keep them from drying out and shrinking. Eggs are produced from what the chicken consumes. Most chickens would not choose corn (cheap filler) if other grains and bugs are available. Be aware if a container indicates an all-vegetable diet, as this often means a lot of corn.

If you are able to find fresh eggs, these are the best. You can check them to see if there is anything unusual inside. Test one by holding it up to a bright light or candle. You'll be able to see any foreign objects, so there is no need to crack it open first.

Energy drinks.

The energy you feel from drinking one of these is caused by unnaturally spiking the glucose for a long period. This is not healthy! The body can only take so many spikes before it revolts. Most all of these drinks contain large amounts of sugar, chemicals, and/or caffeine. Caffeine content can even be hidden in the label under names such as guarana, kola nut, yerba mate and cocoa. Caffeine overdose is often associated with these types of drinks. Studies have shown them to be toxic, and several countries such as Germany, Australia and New Zealand have reported adverse outcomes associated with these drinks: liver damage, kidney failure, respiratory disorders, agitation, confusion, seizures, psychotic conditions, nausea, vomiting, abdominal pain, rhabdomyolysis, tachycardia, cardiac dysrhythmias, hypertension, myocardial infarction, heart failure, and even death. Children, adolescents and young adults are susceptible to cardiac conditions, attention-deficit/hyperactivity, eating disorders and diabetes from these types of beverages.

These beverages interfere with bone mineralization. In children, this is an important point because they are at an important time in skeletal development. The FDA classifies these beverages as dietary supplements, so they are not subject to the same regulations or post-marketing observations that food and soft drinks require. Some manufacturers have chosen to classify their energy drink as a beverage, since the manufacturer is allowed to choose how to categorize and classify their drinks. If it's listed as a beverage, they must self-affirm that the ingredients are "generally safe" for consumption.

Many energy drinks contain added ingredients. When the body's glucose is spiked, insulin is released and the metabolism speeds up. This affects the digestive system by speeding up digestion, making it more difficult to absorb nutrients from healthy food and beverages. These drinks commonly cause dehydration because of this. They are banned in Uruguay, and Canada imposes a caffeine cap. *(www.energydrinkslawsuit.com, Does the FDA Regulate Energy Drinks?)*

Leaving it up to manufacturers to determine how to classify their products and to offer spurious guidance on them is frightening. These beverages, like some sports beverages, are very profitable and not for the health conscious.

Exercise.

Physical activity is vital to health. The body is meant to move. Mobility and muscle mass decrease without exercise. It is difficult for those with disabilities, but without it the body will lose mobility. Exercise can include activities such as home and yard organization and cleaning. Trainers can help, but keep in mind some may not know how to adjust exercise appropriately for those with disabilities, injuries and aging.

Bones need exercise, including the teeth and mouth when chewing. This is where sensible weights can be helpful. Equipment is not necessary; there are creative ways to generate resistance such as lifting gallon water jugs. Find exercise that works for your life-style and is appropriate for your body. There are many protective exercises for the back, the neck, for pregnancy and for older individuals. Walking is one the best and most simple ways to exercise. There is much information out there on how to properly do any exercise, especially lifting.

Get creative. Even dancing around the house is good exercise—and fun! Just make sure the movements are correctly and safely done.

Fasting.

There is a belief that fasting is helpful and healthful. Of course, it depends on the body. When fasting, do not forego proper water hydration. You can live around 45 days without food, but only 3-10 days without water. Kidney damage starts to occur around the third day.

Food fasting does give the body a break, however. It saves energy and rests the digestive system. There are many approaches to fasting. For weight loss, though, fasting requires serious consideration. Some bodies can do just fine with one meal a day.

Some religions, rituals, ceremonies and belief systems involve preset fasting times. The only caveat I have is not hydrating with clean water. Water is more important than food. Dehydration affects how the brain, organs and body function. Regardless of the type of fasting a person chooses, it must be right for that body.

Throughout history, fasting has been a method of attaining enlightenment and great spiritual experiences. After fasting, nutritious food should be introduced slowly, incrementally and in small amounts. If the body is used to eating one meal a day, make it a nutritious meal. An unhealthy meal once a day is wrongly focused. Keeping weight down is great, but it's not necessarily a healthy habit.

Don't entirely avoid hydration until having that once-a-day meal. The amount of liquid taken in during this one meal is hard on the system, raises blood pressure, stretches the stomach and can interfere with saliva. Dehydrating the blood, kidneys and liver for too long is risky.

Fats and Oils.

According to WebMD, roughly 34% to 40% of our calories come from fat. At a minimum, 10% of our calories should come from fat. This is controversial, as some high fat diets are very helpful and considered natural. Seek out guidance as to what your unique body needs.

Fat is necessary for providing nutrients to the brain. Essential fatty acids help keep the skin soft and are needed for the absorption of vitamins and minerals, cell health, blood clotting, muscle movement, heart health, and is also necessary for good energy levels.

Bad fats are saturated, and are solid at room temperature. Good fats are unsaturated, monounsaturated and polyunsaturated. Avoid fake fats, light fats and any fat that insects will not consume such as canola oil. Vegetable oils are considered polyunsaturated, but many of these contain corn oil. Incidentally, rapeseed oil was first used as a mechanical oil.

Hydrogenated fat is unsaturated. Hydrogen acts as a preservative, making the oil more solid and stable so oxygen won't make it rancid. Kitchen oils need to be stored in a tightly closed container to avoid the effects of oxygen.

There are many contradictory studies on what constitutes good fat. Here are a few better ones: avocado oil, walnut oil, sesame oil, grapeseed oil (high heat tolerance), olive oil (low heat tolerance), raw nuts, raw seeds and fish (water pollution content can affect fish oil benefits). Long chain Omega 3 and Omega 6 are in this group and are important to health. *(For more information on Omegas, see the* Supplementation *section below.)* The American heart association recommends at least two servings of fatty fish per week. When nuts and seeds are heated, they convert to bad fat; so raw is always best.

Examples of medium grade fats are partially hydrogenated oil (trans fat), lean red meat, skinless chicken, butter, cheese (not easily digestible), coconut oil (small amounts) and palm oil.

The following are considered to be among the worst (saturated and artificially made): artery clogging trans fats that raise LDL (bad) cholesterol and lower HDL (good), lard, fried foods and processed foods. Fake fat is used to deceive people. It causes vitamin loss, phytochemical loss, digestive upset, anal leakage, has a weird aftertaste, and is more expensive.

Natural is always best. Fake oils like margarine are simply not healthy and likely contain corn. Natural oils should be stored in a cool, dry place. If keeping more than a month, store in the refrigerator. Refining reduces health benefits. Unrefined oils are lightly filtered to remove large particles. Olive oil and sesame oil will look a bit cloudy and have some residue on the bottom if sitting for a while; this is not a concern. Unrefined oils have more intense flavor, are more nutritious and have a shorter shelf life (great for dressings). Ghee is basically butter with the solids removed, and is an excellent alternative to butter.

Some of the information in this section can be confusing. Research and common sense will help. I use real butter and real sour cream in extremely limited amounts, grapeseed oil for sautéing, olive oil in homemade dressings and drizzled on homemade hummus. I also use coconut oil in my skin oil and in cooking. A little goes a long way, so find a balance that works.

There are many ingredients which may not be listed on the labels of fat products. Many contain canola (rapeseed plant) and vegetable oil (mainly corn). In some cases, oil is used to coat the tongue to mask the rotten product used to make the oil.

I buy olive oil from Spain. It is unbelievably different than any I have ever had in the United States. Labeling can be so tricky and inaccurate. Invest in your health, now and in the future, by researching and learning about these things.

There are no fat receptors on the tongue! Fat is used to make items crispy and crunchy, and can aid in lengthening shelf-life from days to months. It also gives more bulk to items like cookies and cakes, which affects how a food feels when bitten. In ground beef, unhealthy saturated fat is considered by the Department of Agriculture to be a nutritional item containing calcium, niacin, iron and others. Ruling organizations must focus on their profits or they would not exist.

Fat is used to cover up and soften the acidic flavor of sour cream, and also aids in enhancing more pleasing flavors. Fat is used very much in processed foods and has a subtle effect on the brain.

Oils can block food nutrients by coating the digestive walls. This interferes with proper absorption at the proper time. In fact, when dipping bread in oil, it actually helps to slow the bread's digestion. Don't dump a ton of healthy, oil-based dressing on a salad. Be light with it so the body can do its work without interference.

Flavorings (natural and artificial).
These can be the most deceiving ingredients on a food label. Many companies add enhancers that cause flavor to pop on the taste buds and dissipate quickly. The purpose is to leave a person unsatisfied and wanting more. If a chemical enhancing flavor contains *any* natural ingredient such as pig-butt oil (enhances the flavor of raspberry), they can label that flavor as natural.

Sweeteners are other flavor enhancing items. The European Union banned Stevia because it interferes with reproduction. Naturally Sweet (Truvia), is a rebiana mix of Stevia and erythritol. Purevia, Zevi, Zerose, and Zsweet are artificial blends of crythritol, a sugar alcohol. Aspartame and sucralose (in all forms) were first developed as insecticides. Stevia and acesulfame K are also sweeteners generally recognized as safe (GRAS). Sucralose seems to be making a comeback, even though it damages 50% of the good bacteria in the intestines.

If possible, use small amounts of raw, unrefined, totally natural sugar, honey, maple, molasses or agave. If you crave any of the previously mentioned fake and questionable sugars, you may be eating and drinking too much of the wrong things. They are all chemical based, either naturally in the plant or through processing. It can be a tough choice for people, especially those addicted to sweet flavors.

Sugar, in any form, should not be more than 15% of your daily calorie intake. A little goes a long way. Get used to eating things without adding sugar. Better to cut back now and avoid its potential conversion to an outright poison which can lead to diseases like diabetes and cancer.

Both natural and unnatural sugars can cause a person to crave more. Putting a sugary syrup on eggs just to get a child to eat them is a tragedy. Learn to enjoy the natural flavors of healthy foods for a longer-lasting and healthy result.

Flour.

Most flour products are absorbed as sugar early in the digestive system. A good alternative is bean or brown rice flour. Grain-based flours lack scientific and physical studies to support their absorbed nutrition value. Flour products should be considered the equivalent of eating junk food.

Sourdough bread is considered the healthiest type due to natural fermentation of the yeast, also known as wild yeast. Some gluten sensitive individuals can get away with eating sourdough bread in limited amounts. Most all store-bought sourdough uses vinegar to impart taste, rather than the traditional use of a starter that forms the fermented natural yeast.

All flour is something that is pulverized, which is very easy for the body to absorb in this form. Flour is absorbed like a sugar in the upper part of the stomach, so the body treats it like sugar. As such, flour is not listed on food labels as a sugar would be. Diets plans that provide prepacked items are often using flour-based products.

A healthier alternative can be Ezekiel bread, which is a sprouted type typically found in the freezer section. Spelt bread can also be a great alternative to traditional bread. Toasting it helps with the flavor and texture.

Fruit.

Fresh fruit is high in fiber and flavor. It is always best to eat as nature has provided. Fruit contains high levels of natural sugar. It is best to eat fruit separately from all other foods. Have some about 20-30 minutes before eating anything else to aid in better absorption of nutrients. Grape skins must be pulverized for best benefits, which makes them great for smoothies. They require chewing thoroughly to break the skins down and to get all the nutrients.

Since fruits are high in sugar, be aware of how much there is in the ones you like. A mango has one of the highest amounts. Just try to balance things out.

Citrus: Most citrus foods are absorbed as an acid. They should be eaten separately, allowing at least 20 minutes before eating anything else. If combined with food, it will cause a frothy mess in the stomach that the body will attempt to force out quickly, leaving no time to absorb much of the food's nutrition.

Lemon and Lime: These are absorbed in the body as an alkaline. They are fine to use with other foods and are great at helping the body get rid of toxins. Be certain to brush your teeth 20 minutes afterward, though. Acid in the mouth has not yet been absorbed in the body as an alkaline and is therefore corrosive to the teeth.

Melons: These are often best to eat separately from all other foods. Otherwise, they could cause gas and digestive issues.

Many fruits are healthy and have great benefits. As with all foods, take things in moderation. The skins often contain the most nutrition. If you want the sweetest and best-tasting one on a tree, look for what the bugs are eating.

Fried foods.

Anything fried is not healthy. Most items are battered in some sort of flour product and dunked in a hot (often chemically created) oil. Studies have shown that arteries to the heart constrict within two hours after eating french fries, lessening blood flow. This amount of fat also coats the intestines, making it extremely hard to absorb any nutrients that may be present.

Frozen foods.

Freezing is an excellent way to stock up on meals. You can make large amounts and freeze them. This is easily done with fresh fruits, soups, chilis, sauces, marinades and meats. It's a great way to deal with leftovers. Prepackaged meals are typically processed, but they are convenient. If you must eat these, try to get ones that are organic or contain low sodium.

Nutritional quality diminishes over time in the freezer. It will vary, depending on altitude and humidity. In general, eat frozen items within three months.

Genetically modified foods.

Modifying foods this way has been common throughout history. A fruit tree can be altered by grafting a cut branch onto a cut branch of another. A fruit farmer may choose tree grafting to boost a fruit's flavor or to modify it. This is different from changing its DNA, a current GMO technique.

Genetically modified foods have less nutrients, less fiber,

and contain many more calories. Bigger food does not mean that it's better. If bugs don't eat it, neither should we.

Many countries have banned GMO foods. America does not require a label to disclose that the food is genetically altered. A DNA-altering component will have an effect on the physical body now and in the future. It's cause and effect.

Gluten.

There is great controversy around this product. Gluten is often used to enhance the texture of bread or its crust, and naturally forms during kneading. Symptoms of gluten sensitivity can include headaches, fatigue, foggy-headedness, disruptive sleep and thyroid issues. Tests do not always reveal a sensitivity, and many professionals refuse to accept that this is a problem.

Gluten free flour is a pulverized item. It gets absorbed as a sugar in the upper part of the stomach. When you must use a flour ingredient, try something that may have at least some benefit such as brown rice. Gluten free does not necessarily mean healthy. Many of these products contain other ingredients that can sabotage health efforts.

Never trust that a restaurant is serving gluten free. Always ask to make sure. If there is any doubt, request a direct answer or that the gluten-free item be brought to you straight from the kitchen.

Grains.

White rice is refined. Get unrefined grains such as barley, quinoa, brown rice and purple rice. As these go through the digestive system, the correct nutrients are extracted at different stages. Grains should never be consumed if chemicals or poison have been placed directly on them. There is no way to keep those toxins from being absorbed into the grain. Many stored grains have this concern because there is competition from hungry rodents. Grains should be a small part of the diet. There is contradiction and controversy over grains. They are fine in limited amounts, but a poor choice as a staple.

Juice.

Organic, unsweetened juices often contain high amounts of sugar. An 8-ounce glass is too much. Drink 2-4 tablespoons at most. It is not normal to eat five oranges or a hundred grapes. Juice should be drunk by itself and not with other items. As mentioned before, a little lemon or lime in water or on food is just fine because it is absorbed as an alkaline rather than an acid. It's ideal to be more alkaline. The typical American breakfast consisting of bread, fried or sautéed potatoes (carbohydrates), eggs and meats (protein) and a big glass of acidic juice does not make nutritional sense.

Juice with added calcium is absurd. Acid breaks down the calcium before it can be used properly in the stomach and intestines. This is just an advertising gimmick with no benefit. Save your money.

Juices can be deceiving. The juice from one orange or tomato is likely less than half a cup. If you drink juice, don't drink more than the yield of one item. With large fruits, like grapefruit, stick with the same half cup or less. Juices are high in sugar and calories, and they lack important fiber. It's always better to eat the original item rather than its juice.

Organic, pure cranberry juice has benefits for the bladder. It has no added sugar, so it's somewhat bitter. Cranberry juice can benefit those who struggle with their bladder and are sensitive to infections. Be sure you are also getting enough water daily.

Grape juice has some benefits, but the majority of nutrients are in the grape skin, not the juice.

Tomato juice is highly acidic and should be kept to a minimum (like any juice). One tomato does not contain 10 ounces of juice. This is also true for tomato sauces. Counter with a lot of leafy and above-ground vegetables.

Meat.

Some people require meat and some do not. Bodies change over time and often require less of this protein later on. Some will need to eliminate it entirely. The first meat to eliminate should be pork, then beef, bison, chicken and other fowl. Fish is meant to be a supporter of life. Most will be fine with foods from the ocean. As spiritual development evolves, meat protein from animals that walk the earth can become a hindrance.

Farm raised fish are exposed to pollution runoffs on the land. Other animals are fed steroids and killed before they die of anemia. Some stores use outrageous practices to sell meat that is nearing (or past) its expiration date. They wash it off, pump fake red watery substances into it, or pile on seasonings to disguise its worn condition.

Wild caught fish is always the best type, but beware: They can be easily replaced with much cheaper fish—even ones that are not digestible—and the purchaser has no idea. It's also easier to hide when fried or covered in sauces. Some unscrupulous restaurants have used this to their advantage.

Animals raised too close to each other without real movement is not natural. This is why so many antibiotics are used to keep animals from making each other sick or dying off. Hormones are pumped into them to make them grow abnormally fast. Animals are slaughtered before they die of anemia and lack of nutrients, lest their meat become more contaminated for consumption. Meat is not nutritious this way. It can cause all sorts of human issues such as iron or protein deficiencies.

If you have ever eaten stringy-like chicken, most likely it was pumped with growth hormones. All meat should spring back when you gently push on it. If it is mushy, avoid it.

Fear affects taste and texture. Some companies buy directly from compassionate farms and ranches that treat and manage the animals humanely. It makes a difference, even though it costs much more because of this.

Mushrooms.

Mushrooms contain antioxidants (selenium, vitamin C, choline), small amounts of calcium, minerals, protein, a tiny amount of vitamin D, fiber and potassium. There are many kinds and the nutrients vary. Mushrooms must be cooked for the nutrients to be absorbable. Some kinds, like portabella, can be a substitute for meat. A portabella sandwich is a lovely treat. They are also low in calories.

Nuts.

Edgar Cayce recommended 3-5 raw almonds a day to keep cancer away. There is no need to eat a handful or dozens of nuts; only a few are needed. Once a nut is roasted or cooked, the oil becomes a bad oil. There are also ridiculous amounts of salt and oil that get added to them. The exception is peanuts. Although the oil becomes bad when heated, it is a tradeoff to peanuts containing goitrogen *(see Thyroid section)*. Skip the bread and eat no more than a teaspoon or two once in a while.

Some studies advise to soak nuts and seeds in clean water for at least eight hours before consuming and to discard remainders after 48 hours. Nuts contain a non-digestible component called phytic acid (phytates), which can bind with minerals and can contain enzyme inhibitors, These are released when soaking. Some even add salt to aid in drawing out unwanted items, then rinse it off before drying.

Using nuts to make almond milk usually involves just water and the nuts. Drinking a beverage that contains around 50 nuts is not normal. It is high in calories and heavily watered down. Chewing is the first step in proper digestion. Don't waste good nutrients this way.

In the United States, manufactured nuts must be sprayed with an antibacterial product unless they come directly from a farm. The product usually remains on them for a couple of minutes, yet companies claim none of the toxins get absorbed. This is pasteurization. Get unpasteurized organic nuts directly from the farms.

Unpasteurized raw almonds, pecans and walnuts are wonderful. Unpasteurized raw cashews are a nice treat from time to time. Keep nuts in the refrigerator in a tight and covered container to help with freshness.

These are easy and light enough to carry in a baggie in a pocket, briefcase or purse. Having a healthy, protein rich snack can help get you through when you need to.

Organic.

Toxins are everywhere. Limiting them where we can will assist the body in maintaining its marvelous ability to flush unavoidable toxins. The preferred order of organic significance is dairy, meats, vegetables, fruits, then processed foods. Farm fresh sources and farmers markets can be good alternatives. Some offer organic items and chicken eggs (from their chickens) that freely roam and eat bugs and seeds rather than cheap corn.

With illness, the body must endure life stresses and adaptations. Health should be a high priority. Without it, life has far less joy. Cheap food is cheap for a reason. Those who fool the public by falsely claiming something is organic are just overcharging. We should use our dollars where integrity is consistent. Positive change can occur!

Be wary of some stores that carry organic items for a while, then slowly pull them off the shelf to influence customers into going back to non-organic. There are many tactics used, but you have power with the dollar.

Processed food.

Nature is always best. Limit processed foods such as flour products, chain restaurants, fast food, canned, prepackaged and prepackaged frozen items as much as possible. Eat simply rather than having lots of sauces, gravy, salt, sugar, and other add-ons. Know what is in your food and who has handled it. Many foods are amazing in their original state, like fresh beets and raw cashews. Consider trying natural items before getting processed ones.

Protein.

Protein is essential to health. It is found in a variety of foods such as meat, seafood, hemp, dairy, eggs, beans, nuts, whole grains and many vegetables. For a sedentary average woman, 46 grams daily is recommended. For a sedentary average man, it's 56 grams. It is suggested that a person get two 3-ounce servings of meat per day. There are alternatives to meat, such as jack fruit, that can be helpful in meeting proteins needs.

There are many ways to get protein, and it should be spread throughout the day. Although soy is low in fat and high in protein, it is scientifically proven to be connected to thyroid disease *(see Thyroid section).*

Whey protein isolate, pumpkin seed powder and hemp protein are good protein alternatives. Mix it up and try not to get stuck having the same thing over and over. Hemp seeds are naturally sweet and very tasty. Sprinkle some on oatmeal to boost protein. Pea protein is linked to gout. If there is a genetic predisposition to gout in your family, you may want to avoid this one.

Salt.

All natural, high-altitude sea salt is one of the best types. I use pink Himalayan sea salt. Regular table salt with added sodium contains a non-clumping ingredient to keep it from clumping before use. Unfortunately, this causes the salt to get stuck in the body, causing salt buildup there. This can directly affect weight and blood pressure. The body is capable of flushing sea salt out daily. In order to flush table salt, one needs to take in only *clean* water for three days to begin its release. Salt is addictive and should be used sparingly.

Read the food labels. Soup-based items, for example, are extremely high in sodium.

Limit all salt. It alters natural flavor and is not necessary in most cases. When a person stops eating so many salty items, their taste buds will return to normal, enhancing the flavor of nutritious nature-made items.

Many items contain salt, especially in processed or restaurant foods. In bars and restaurants, salt is often used to subtly trigger people into wanting more beverages and food. It increases appetite and thirst. It's also used in prepared weight-loss items in hopes that a person will eat more. Salt comes in many forms, and food labels may not fully disclose how much is really in a product. Without salt, processed foods would no longer exist.

Soy.

As mentioned earlier, soy should be highly limited. Soybean, edamame and soybean meal (fed to animals) should all be considered. Soy is a main staple of certain cultures, but we should reconsider its role as we learn more about it. As mentioned in the Thyroid section, soy blocks iodine to this gland *(see Goitrogen section).*

Starchy foods.

Avoid too many starchy foods if you are trying to lose weight. Although some have health benefits, most do not. Starchy foods include flour products, bananas, bread, chips, garlic, nuts, oatmeal, pasta, popcorn, potatoes, squashes, tapioca, rice and corn. Gravies, sauces, store bought dressings and toppings are usually full of starch, sugar, fat, salt and/or chemicals.

Sugar.

Eliminate high sugar items. If you have reached your desired weight goal, add them back in small amounts. Beets, carrots, honey, fruits, maple syrup and molasses should be used only on occasion and in limited amounts. Over the course of a day, sugared and floured items can add up quickly. Refer to the Flavorings section above for more information on sugar.

There is a "bliss point" in the food industry. This is a taste threshold where sugar can cause a repulsive reaction on the tongue if it crosses the bliss point. It is used very much to the advantage of profiteers. Sugar adds up quickly because natural and fake sugars, along with processed items, all become sugar in the body. It is highly addictive and gets snatched up by the brain. The body grabs it from there, leaving the brain wanting more.

Among many wonderful books on the subject, Michael Moss's book, *Salt, Sugar, Fat,* is an excellent consult. It is worth educating yourself on the facts and truths about these substances.

In summary, drastically limit sugar. Avoid adding it to anything and avoid addictive sugary items; they contain no nutrition. Don't waste your time on this nasty *carboplunk.* Think nutrition!

Supplementation.

Supplementation is controversial, but people consistently do this when dealing with a health issue. Keep in mind that too much of anything becomes bad, so variety and its absorbability are most important.

When supplementing, I use non-GMO based items from

sea vegetables, vegetable derived vitamins and minerals, Omega-3's and 6's, and some sort of calcium such as grass-fed bone capsules (chelated is fine). I also include vitamin C from rosehips—not ascorbic acid. My supplements are mostly organic vegetables and/or fruits. There is no need to consume every day, as the body needs to be surprised once in a while.

Omega-3's and 6's are mainly linoleic acid. Omega-3's fatty acid contains EPA and DHA, which are abundant in fish and marine life. These are necessary for brain function and thinking, and are important for vision and normal development of organs. Omega-3 acids become a hormone-like substance which aids the heart and immune system. Omega-6 acids play a big part in body functionality. They protect cells in the body; however, there is much better benefit from natural foods. Wild salmon is easy to cook and highly nutritious. Studies show that Omega capsules alone, over time, are not as healthy as they seem. Try to get your Omegas from real sources. If you must supplement, mix it up and don't take them every single day.

If a person consumes fish, nuts, seeds, healthy vegetables, oils, sea vegetables and a little grain, they are likely getting enough Omega-6. Ten ounces of healthy fish per week provides the needed Omega-3's and 6's. It is recommended that for every one fatty acid Omega-3 there should be four fatty acid Omega-6's. However, too much may increase damage caused by the natural oxidization of cells. Keep in mind that this type of supplementation uses fish liver and fish skins.

The liver and skins of animals (and seal oil) contain toxins such as concentrated pesticides, heavy metals and other contaminants found in the ocean. They can also contain high levels of vitamins A and D. With chicken, the skin has benefits for an ill person, but most the time it's just added fat. A little goes a long way.

If someone feels the need to take vitamin B supplements, do NOT take the B-12 kind that starts with "cyan". These contain cyanide (used to bind the two molecules that make up the vitamin), which speeds up metabolism. This is the reason a person feels energized after taking this type. The body speeds up in order to get rid of the poison in the system. In studies, very little (if any) of the B vitamin is absorbed from this type, either sublingually, by pill or by shot (which only benefits if very deficient).

Studies show that some over-the-counter supplementation may not even get broken down, so the pills get pooped out without being absorbed. They can contain sugar, colorings, flavorings and unnecessary chemicals. Pulverized mineral rocks in non-vegetable-derived supplements are not absorbable.

Use all-vegetable derived vitamins and minerals. For example, if taking D3, lessen your calcium intake because it aids in calcium absorption. Get your vitamin C from rosehips, not ascorbic acid.

Take breaks with supplementation. This way, the body does not get lazy in its ability to take in nutrients naturally. It also gives the body a chance to balance, and helps people be more attentive to what they are eating. Check with your doctor and a skilled nutritionist trained beyond the Western approaches. Some supplements such as vitamin A thin the blood and can cause complications.

If facing a health crisis, a surgery or taking blood thinners, talk to a professional about VitaMedica products, which are designed for such things. They offer before, during and after-surgery vitamins that promote health and healing without risking complications. These can aid in speeding up the healing and help with bruising. Quality cosmetic surgeons are a great resource for this supplement, as they are the ones who often recommend them to their patients.

Vegetables.

The body needs vegetables, especially dark leafy greens. Vegetables are healing! Without them, you hinder the body tremendously. Lettuce can be eaten by itself; in fact, it's easy to grab a leaf, munch it down and move on. Very little dressing is needed, so you can limit this topping. Try sautéing diced onions with red peppers and placing them hot on the salad. Some people can handle these in smoothies, but some cannot. I'm a believer in using super-dehydrated vegetable mixes in my smoothies 2 to 3 times a week. Avoid as much as possible those that have Stevia or other sweeteners.

A rule of thumb ratio is to eat three above-ground vegetables to one below-ground. The majority of those below ground are high in starch and sugar.

Peas have a connection to gout, so that's something to consider. Once in a while is fine, though. Most of the time, the body can handle it. In this case, it may not be worth the risk when there are so many others to choose from.

Variety is the key. Mix it up and try new vegetables. Keep the body guessing by it not expecting the same old vegetables. Be careful what you put on vegetables, though. Adding a bunch of butter, salt and other enhancers can turn your healthy choice into a bad choice.

Lightly cooking vegetables makes it easier on the digestive system. Raw is great if the body can handle it. When illness hits, make things easier to digest by cooking them. The key here is a wide variety. Keep it simple and avoid adding too many spices, sugars or sauces.

Water and hydration.
Our bodies are 70% water and they need hydration. Clean, purified water is the best. Some bodies need more than others, some are fine with less. The environment also contributes to the amount of hydration needed. Don't compare your intake levels with others. If your skin and lips become dry or your nose often runs, you may need more hydration. Clearing the throat, itching and red patches can also be signs. Parents should highly consider water as a default beverage for their children from very young until grown. Lead by example. Avoid adding anything like sugar or milk to any beverage. Many beverages already contain high amounts of sugar, flavoring and colorings which aid in addicting people.

Start the day with a cup or so of water after cleaning the mouth and before anything else. This helps to flush toxins from the kidneys, which have been working throughout the night to detoxify. Avoid drinking a lot of water before or with meals. Large amounts are harmful and stretch out the stomach.

Wrapping Up

Variety and moderation in all things are the golden keys. Do the research and keep in mind that studies can easily result in conclusions that suit the Security Profitability Formula.

Pay attention to the body's sensations and emotions that rise up, as these are guides to what is working and what may not be the best choice. Everything requires wisdom and spiritual guidance.

Attitude is everything! Love your amazing body. Correct anything that does not support it. Be determined to live your life feeling as amazing and energetic as possible. It is a lifestyle, not a fad or temporary fix. Feeling amazing is better than anything. Why wait until health is damaged or lost to create change? Be the ruler of your body universe with honesty, respect, compassion and healthy supportive actions.

7| Tips and Tricks

Modern humans do not usually get the exercise they used to. Some sciences also hinder efforts towards health, as they can be influenced by others and refuse to evolve when new knowledge emerges. The effects of the modern diet on tribes around the world is profound. There is no argument that high amounts of sugar, flour and other *carboplunks* destroy health. In these modern times, you must also be concerned about the amount of toxins in, on and around the body. When the liver gets overloaded with toxins, it shoots them out into the blood stream for the kidneys to handle. The organs are not designed to handle such an overload. The body and mind need help.

Most people eat way too much, often because of boredom. Find some activities and keep hydrated with clean water. Find ways to counter the Secure Profitability Formula. Here are some considerations:

Starting the day.

Before getting out of bed, set your attitude and intent for the day. This just takes a couple of minutes. Start with your mind directed toward health and success. Be realistic. There are many affirmations, prayers, meditations and mantras that can help you design what is perfect for your needs. Here's an outline that supports your intent:

- Today, I will only put healthy items in my mouth.
- I will do this by being prepared and making sure I have some items easily available to me.
- Throughout the day, I will remind myself of this goal.
- I will not do anything that does not fit this goal.
- All choices are to support a healthy body and mind.
- I love and believe in myself and my choices.
- I remind my brain that it is serving my goals and to let go of outside influences that do not serve my goals.

Don't lounge around in bed. Get up and get moving. Force yourself to get ready for the day, make the bed and get out of your night clothes, even if you have the day off. Otherwise, it promotes laziness.

If you feel rushed, set the alarm a bit earlier. Shut off the television. Do a small meditation, prayer, mantra or visualization. Have a routine so the body knows what is about to happen and can support you.

You should be able to enjoy a beverage or a moment to yourself without feeling rushed. Providing yourself with a few moments can be a wonderful opportunity for creating calmness for the day. Getting the mind, body and spirit on the same page is a recipe for success. Meditation, prayer or setting an intention will do that. You are much more apt to handle any challenge with clarity and ease. Life will always have twists and turns. You are meant to be adaptable and flexible without getting bent out of shape.

Life is all about solving problems and moving on. When expectations are disrupted, it can cause a person to react like a spoiled child. Learn to go with it instead of against it. Find out how you can help move things forward for everyone. Problems are solved by being aware, alert and out of your head. Don't try so hard. Be in the moment so you can be alert. If the thinking isn't working, change it. If you cannot change it, ask for help.

Weight is an ongoing struggle for those influenced by the Western diet. Here are some tips I found very helpful for losing and maintaining appropriate weight for my body:

Calories count.

Keep the body guessing. Nutrition is what you are after. Weight is an issue for most people. The goal is to be at a healthy weight for your body. If you are well-hydrated, be aware of the amount and types of nutrition you provide the body.

Sugar calories from *carboplunks* are different than those from real foods like fruits. A tablespoon of sugar has similar calories as a medium sized apple. The apple is denser with other nutrients and fiber, and satisfies hunger much longer. The sugar is just empty calories. Refined (or processed) sugars have many names such as white sugar, brown sugar, cane sugar, coconut sugar, palm, invert, high-fructose corn syrup and more. Although these are often from plants they have been processed. They are added to foods, often to the bliss point, to help with taste and food preservation. It lacks nutrition. Most fruit is 40-55% fructose, compared to table sugar at 50% fructose and 50% glucose. Fructose, which gets broken down in the liver, often ends up as fat in the body. The body is capable of maintaining proper levels, but it takes longer for the body to process fructose. Glucose is broken down in the stomach and needs insulin to get into the bloodstream before it can be broken down. Sugar is simply not good for the body but the nutrients in the fruit are. This is why it is not healthy to eat too many fruits. Fruits are not the only items that contain sugar.

Fruits with the lowest sugar content are; raspberries, blackberries, and strawberries. Those highest are dried fruits, bananas, and mangoes. Fruit juice also tends to be high in sugar. Items like flour get absorbed early on in the upper stomach and are just sugar to the body. Drastically limit items like flours and those with high refined sugars. Keep a watch on the type of sugar calories you are consuming.

Start your day out with clean water to flush the kidneys, and drastically limit caffeine and teas. The body requires clean water the most. Afterward, wait about 15 minutes before that first cup of coffee or tea—not a mug, but a cup. In fact, get rid of caffeine or at least take breaks from it. It may be difficult because it is addictive and easy to get used to.

One of my favorite morning beverages is 1-2 tablespoons of honey combined with 1-2 teaspoons of Ceylon cinnamon in a cup of hot water. This is better than coffee and will perk you up. The honey is antibacterial and the cinnamon is spicy and does not dissolve. The spice excites the capillaries in the mouth and throat, and the cinnamon cleans the veins as it travels through the blood. It also curbs appetite. Have one to three of these drinks per day, but not at bedtime. Check with your doctor if you are diabetic.

For a detoxifying beverage, try half a lemon in hot water. Add a touch of cayenne pepper for a lift. Be sure to wait 20 minutes before brushing the teeth.

Here's another one. Mix ½ to 1 teaspoon of unflavored gelatin in a small amount of juice, in a smoothie or other room-temperature or cool liquid. This increases the absorption of vitamins and aids the glands and various organs.

Sometimes the body needs a bit of nourishment in the morning. A few nuts, a piece of fruit, or even water with a soluble super dehydrated fruit and vegetable mix can be incredible. I like the Greens First brand. It contains Stevia (a sweetener that should only be used in very small quantities), which gives it a nice sweet flavor. I plop a scoop in a 16-ounce water container, shake it and go. It's a great way to get a burst of nutrients with hydration. I will do this any time of day, but not every day.

Raise Blood Sugar without Spiking Glucose:

- 1-2 Tablespoons Concord Grape Juice
- 1-2 Tablespoons Water

Sometimes when losing weight, the body is not used to the change in calories. It may go into starvation mode, which is when you feel super hungry and might shake a little, because the blood sugar is too low. When this happens, the body will take anything you give it and convert it to fat. It is a natural means of keeping the body safe. The beverage above will stem the starvation mode and give you a bit of time to make healthier choices. It is a nice go-to for losing weight. If you wake up in the middle of the night feeling hungry, it calms things down so you can get right back to sleep. It can also be used half an hour before a meal to curb the appetite. Try this before going to a restaurant so you can make healthier choices.

When eating at a restaurant, make choices that serve your goals. There is no need to eat a full meal. A salad, soup or a side can all be chosen instead of a full meal. It may be difficult, but avoid bread to start the meal. There is no reason to eat a full restaurant serving. Water is the best beverage, but keep in mind it is likely from the faucet (tap) and not filtered. When having salad, get the dressing on the side so you can control the amount. The tip and front edges of the tongue perceive salty or sweet, depending on the diagram you are looking at. The area behind that perceives sweet or salty. Put the salad on your fork, then dip the tip in the dressing. This way, you get the flavor of the dressing without using much. Consider eating part of the salad "as is" before using dressing. Also, avoid additional items like croutons or sesame sticks.

Cheap Tomato Beverage:

- 2 Tablespoons Tomato Paste
- 1 cup hot water
- A pinch of onion powder, garlic powder and sea salt

This drink is filling, somewhat tasty, curbs the appetite and has about 30 calories. It's also acidic, so be sure to balance it out later with appropriate vegetables. It is not as tasty as real soup, but it works.

Bone broth.

Find real bone broths rather than bullion and soup presented as bone broth. This one is great on occasion. It is also inexpensive to make your own broth and freeze it for future use. They are easy to find online. Some bones can easily be picked up from the meat department or butcher.

Smoothies.

This is a great way to add nutrition, protein and fiber with decent calories. The more high-sugar fruits are used, the higher the calories. Only a small amount of fruit is needed. Fruit helps the flavor. Juice is naturally high in calories, so don't use much if you go this route. I mix it up and drink these when I am losing weight, to add a punch of nutrition and to help get me back on track. It is a great energy booster, and the body responds positively.

Get a super dehydrated fruit and vegetable mix. I occasionally use the Orgain Organic Superfoods berry flavor for added taste. Add a touch of Garden of Life Raw Organic Perfect Food, an alkalizer and detoxifier. Next, add a bit of pure unflavored Kosher protein, pasture-raised and grass-fed collagen hydrolysate to aid the joints. Lily of the Desert is a mild aloe vera. I use the inner fillet and about 2 tablespoons to the mixture. Aloe has many nutrients and benefits.

Use a good amount of clean water and a bit of fruit to make this less earthy tasting and easier to drink. I use a straw because it makes it easier for me to drink. Don't use too much fruit. Find a happy medium where it's just enough to help the flavor. My favorite fruits to use are fresh or frozen pineapple, mango, apple, blueberries, peaches, plums, grapes, kiwi and pears. On occasion, I might use bananas or add a tablespoon or so of cranberry or grape juice. When you choose your fruits, always be aware of the sugar content.

Try a bit of pumpkin seed protein powder, but not every time. There are certain healthy thresholds, so mix it up. Hemp protein powder is an excellent choice, unsweetened and organic with maximum fiber.

Calories can add up. If I make more than 8-10 ounces, I store the extra in the refrigerator for later or the next day. It can be between 300-600 calories depending on what you are adding and if consuming more than 10 ounces. Remember to swirl these beverages around in the mouth to allow the saliva enzymes to do their work.

The above smoothie will increase energy, help shrink the stomach and get the body used to having less food. It was designed to be a full meal replacement with high nutrition and equal or lower calories. You will feel amazing after just a couple of these. It is not designed for long-term everyday use, though. You want the body to do its work by absorbing nutrients from real food. Don't get lazy with such an easily absorbed drink. Take a break, then repeat.

Limit or eliminate alcoholic beverages, caffeine, sugar, teas, sodas or any carbonated drinks (very hard on the digestive system), processed cocoa, ground flour products and corn.

Sourdough bread.

The majority of sourdough bread in the stores are made with vinegar and not wild yeast. I do make my own sourdough bread. It takes a bit of effort initially and too big of a subject to cover here. In brief, flour and water are used to build a wonderful natural yeast. There is some waste involved while the yeast is maturing and gaining great flavor. Mine took about 2 months and is very strong and medium in sour flavor. I kept it in the refrigerator after that and fed (necessary to keep the healthy bacteria alive) once a week and make a loaf of bread once every week or two. The science behind this is very cool. In short, the mixture grabs the healthy bacteria from the air and it creates the yeast. Like anything live it must be fed and properly maintained.

After two years, I dehydrated a bunch of it, along with some rye based wild yeast, and no longer keep ongoing undehydrated. I take 1 teaspoon of the dehydrated small pieces and in about 4 days of feeding I can then make 2 loafs of bread, or 1 loaf with rolls, crackers, jalapeno/cheese, or whatever I am choosing to do. To make real artesian bread, which is wonderfully incredible, it will require 2 full pages of steps and 2 days to make. I have done this only a couple times. I much prefer a simple country loaf made from the sourdough starter because it is easier.

Sourdough freezes great but does not refrigerate well. I have limited freezer space so do not let it rise very tall. After cooling the freshly baked bread, I slice in thin slices (a way to limit my intake of a flour-based product) and freeze. When I want a slice I just pop one off, defrost, warm up or toast. For rolls I wrap them individually in plastic wrap and put in a freezer bag. I then can grab one, defrost and warm it up. This way I always have a bit of bread around but don't have to use it up or eat it consistently. I generally go through about

2 loafs at most every 3 months which is how long it lasts in the freezer.

Wild yeast can be used for many things and there is a lot of information out there. In figuring this out for myself I did gravitate towards trained chefs for initial instruction. I then found a book that had many different recipes and went from there. Do not believe you must waste a ton of it the starter. Wild yeast is stronger than many realize and a little can go a long way. What I find amazing is that I do not gain weight eating this bread. Commercial bread causes quick weight gain. I rarely eat more than one slice. It is very filling, and the flour I use is a higher-protein organic bread and all-purpose flour.

Real sourdough has many benefits. It has lots of nutrients and healthy carbs, protein, fiber and vitamins, but it is still flour-based. It improves digestion, lowers chronic disease risk, and promotes healthy aging due to the wild yeast that is used. Its nutrients are easily absorbed and acts as a prebiotic (helps to feed the good bacteria in the intestines). It is lower in gluten due to it not being kneaded as much as other bread. Some people who are sensitive to gluten can get away with eating it, but I do not advise this as the body does not want gluten.

The use of wild yeast is ancient and how our ancestors were able to make flour type products. It also helps to avoid buying such things like crackers because the homemade are so amazing that commercial doesn't even come close. Choose a recipe book that gives many options for using the yeast.

There are also many places to purchase real wild yeast like this, but you must do your research. They often do the same by dehydrating it. Some live wild yeasts may be hundreds of years old.

Not everyone can do such things but for me it has been totally worth learning and doing. Now that I have several quarts dehydrated, it will last me many years and makes it less expensive and easy.

Sprouted breads.

Sprouted breads like Ezekiel can be a great alternative. They are made from whole grains that have begun to sprout or germinate. Sprouting partially breaks down the starch in the grains (34 grams in a 4-ounce serving compared to 44 grams in a 12-grain bread). It also has higher fiber content and a low glycemic index. Due to the sprouts containing water, the calorie count in the bread is lower. You can find it in the freezer department, and it's often best to serve toasted. My favorites are the English muffin and cinnamon swirl. It is a nice change of pace, convenient and another healthy alternative.

Fruit vinegars.

Fruit vinegars are super easy to make. Store-bought fruit vinegar, however, is simply not real. It is typically white vinegar with a splash or two of juice. Raisin, organic blueberry (from frozen) and organic mango (from frozen) are good to make. These are easy to find the process and can be a bit tricky the first time. There is much information on this process, as well as some environmental considerations. Vinegars can last years before being consumed.

A splash of raisin vinegar on freshly sautéed vegetables adds amazing flavor. The mango makes a great salad dressing by adding a touch of honey or making some into a habanero mango BBQ sauce. I like to splash a touch of the blueberry in cool water for a detoxifying start to my day.

In this process, the fruit becomes alcohol based, then becomes vinegar. I have not made apple cider vinegar, but it will be the next one I try since it is such a common ingredient in my kitchen.

Weight loss.

To find out if you need to lose some weight, try the sternum check. The sternum is located just below the chest where the ribs come together. When this begins to pooch out, the heart is covered in fat cells. The fat has no place else to go but outward. This is the same for the rest of the abdomen. The body cavity gets so full of fat that it must push the tummy out to accommodate more. Also, if your breasts sit on top of your tummy when you sit, you have too much fat. Body size and age must also be considered. This is just a guide. It's about a healthy weight that works for your body and you.

Most people struggle with this. If you keep an eye on the sternum, it can be easier to resolve before anything gets out of hand. Turn sideways in the mirror and check yourself. Look at the distance from the front of the abdomen to the back of the bum. Too often, the truth can be missed looking from the front view only. If your clothes don't fit well, you have gained weight. Don't use undergarments that squish and bind to hide and reshape the body. These block healthy lymph from flowing, disrupt circulation and breathing, cause back and pectoral muscles to weaken, disrupt digestion, and can also deform the rib cage. A healthy weight is different for everyone and it depends on many factors. Unnecessary weight has many risks and makes it hard on the joints. It tells you right away that you are eating too much or too many of the wrong foods. You are not alone, and there is much you can do to become a healthier you.

If the body says *enough*, stop and do something about it. People come in many shapes and sizes. It's all good unless it affects your health. Faking appearance by hurting the body, like using garments that squish the body, is not good for you. Learn your shape and where and how you gain weight. It is annoying for someone to suggest to a person who watches their weight that they can eat anything they want. It is often not true.

Genetics must also be considered. If there is a family history of diabetes, obesity or other weight related issues, you might choose to be more aware and take action early before any issues arise. Not everyone is meant to live a slender life. Real people are accepting and understanding. Do what you can and don't beat yourself up. This can be difficult with a family or partner who has no interest in being healthy, but you have a choice whether or not to give in to that. This is not a new issue and is common. Get help to figure out how to think and stay on track for yourself. Using kind words like "no" or "no thanks" in a soft tone with no explanation can do wonders. There is no reason to explain yourself. Keep smiling and avoid negative emotions. This is a personal health choice.

Those of us with injuries and challenges must be even more vigilant. Adding pressure to injured joints, ligaments and muscles only creates more issues. Proper nutrition curbs hunger; *carboplunks* add to hunger. The body craves healthy nutrition. Give your body time to adjust to new thinking and actions.

There will be times when the body hits a set point. This is a weight it has experienced before and was comfortable with. It may take a little time for the body and brain to realize you are losing weight before it gets past this set point and heads to the next. Be patient and allow the body and mind to catch up. They are designed to support you, and they will with a little patience and understanding.

Learn to thrive despite the chaos all around you. Be healthy, make wise and caring choices and adapt to changes. Joy will increase naturally. Keep moving and keep learning. Think and act in healthy, loving ways.

Being more self-sufficient.

The cost of living is skyrocketing and the quality of commercial foods and pre-prepared items continues to decline. Relying on others to plan, prepare, serve and clean is risky. This approach can be costly. A restaurant must make a profit despite increasing food costs and short shelf lives. I love the restaurant experience, but want to know the quality of the food and what's in it.

It is not by accident that so many people don't plan, prep and cook for themselves—not to mention the added health risks and medical and pharmaceutical support that come from high cholesterol, salt/sodium, sugar, chemicals and saturated fats.

The only way to combat this is to become more self-sufficient and learn how to do these things yourself. It is not cheaper to eat out than in, even with discounts and coupons.

The health damage is very costly. Humans are easily conditioned and manipulated. It's up to you to take charge.

There are many ways to make simple meals and learn as you go. Learn how to meet this daily need in healthy ways. It does not have to be complicated, nor does it require a lot of spices and ingredients. Keep it simple.

Shopping and Other Tips

I have met many people from other countries who have commented on the low quality of American fruits and vegetables. The food from many countries is organic and much better quality. There are exceptions, but in general, it's a sad statement about our country.

I choose organic most of the time, even though it may or may not be what I really get. The only way to truly know is to grow your own food. The following will highlight basic info on what people purchase and use.

Citrus: Choose smoother skin and fewer deep dimples. Lemons and limes lend a shine due to the oils in their skins. These are juicy fruits compared to drier, deep dimpled and older ones.

Dairy: Use whole milk, not lite. Buttermilk is great for baking and for the occasional ranch dressing, and has less calories than milk. Also try real and unsalted butter. Most fakes contain unhealthy oils and chemicals. Always choose one with the furthest expiration date. Most dairy freezes really well, even yogurt. If it curdles when defrosted, just whisk it up and it will smooth out. Marinades based in dairy also freeze well.

Eggs: These should be even in color, clean and similar in size without a bunch of specks. There should be no damage to the shells. Fresh hen eggs do not need refrigeration for up to four weeks, but you can if you wish. Surprisingly, it is not advised to wash fresh eggs. Just wipe them off and they will last even longer. Washing removes the bloom (cuticle), which is the protective coating on the shell. This keeps bacteria from getting through to the egg inside. Commercial eggs are coated with mineral oil after washing to help with this. Do not wash eggs before use, even if commercial, as this can push bacteria into the egg. If eggs have been refrigerated, I find it best to continue refrigeration. Do not use eggs with a broken shell. Once cooked, refrigerate. When boiling eggs, you can use a steamer, place them in cold water and peel right away before they cool. Store in the refrigerator in a container with a wet paper towel on the bottom to keep the eggs from drying out. There are several ways to store boiled eggs.

Egg shells are excellent sources of calcium. If you boil your eggs, save the water, let it cool and pour into the soil of your plants. Crunch the leftover shells and spread them on the lawn and around garden plants. There are many great uses and benefits.

Farmer markets.

Not all of these sellers are genuine. Do some research or drive by a farm to make sure it really exists. Healthy efforts are worth knowing the truth. I loved going to the farmers market when I was near one. I based my weekly menu on finding the best fruits and vegetables at the market. Some also offer quality seafood and meats.

Fats.

Some fats such as grape seed oil, avocado oil, coconut oil and olive oil have high temperature tolerances. If any oil gives off smoke, that smoke is toxic and should be avoided. When an oil reaches its temperature limit, it becomes a bad, unhealthy oil.

I use grape seed oil for cooking, and quality olive and avocado oils in dressing and for drizzles. Coconut oil is very high in calories, so a little goes a long way. I also make skin and scalp oils from it. I find olive oil best for dressings and for drizzling on lightly cooked vegetables and hummus.

Many oils have other unlisted and unwanted oils in them. Consider buying olive oil directly from Spain and other countries that do not use GMO and hidden ingredients. The price is certainly higher, but you get what you pay for. This is one benefit to online shopping.

Using too much oil (as in frying) coats the lining of the intestinal tract and blocks the absorption of nutrients.

General fruit.

Extra-large fruit is usually genetically altered with higher calories and less fiber. It is the nutrient and fiber content you are after, not the size. When selecting fruit, be sure to check freshness and for any bruising or mold. Apples should be firm, and at certain times of the year they are sweeter. Pineapple should have a bit of yellow around it, and the bottom center should not be dried out. Try new fruits and research their nutrition level. Don't get stuck using the same fruit over and over. Surprise the body!

Pomegranate is delicious and has many health benefits.

The pre-packaged arils (seeds with juice sacks) can be expensive, but they are fully eatable and have great fiber. This fruit is easy to slice and separate. It's a bit messy, but so delicious.

Kiwi is like a big grape. It can be eaten with or without the skin; however, I peel them because the fuzzy skin texture does not appeal to me. The peel easily blends into a smoothie, and the additional fiber and nutrients are a good thing.

I keep dehydrated mango for easy snacks and dehydrated blueberries for topping my salads. Three pounds of frozen blueberries will fit into a pint jar after dehydrating. They are like raisins and aren't soaked with sugar. I also keep prunes, which are filling, in the refrigerator. In-season fruits are usually fresher than those shipped in from elsewhere.

You can even arrange to buy directly from the farmers. Instead of sitting in front of the television, take a field trip one day and learn about the local fruits.

Herbs and spices.

Fresh is always a great choice, but often not practical. Spice containers may also contain unnecessary fillers. Spices are necessary to boost flavors, though. In particular, some spices like Mexican spices are best sautéed in a touch of oil before mixing into a food to bring out the flavor. In fact, putting such spice mixtures together beforehand can be great fun. It teaches children how to measure and shows what usually goes into such mixtures. Spices can also be medicinal. It's pretty easy to grow basil, rosemary and parsley. Each has many uses. Find ways that work well for you.

Things that are dehydrated have a good shelf life. If the spice is a bit old, just add more. If they are kept in a dark cool place, they can last a for a long time. If buying spices in bulk, choose those you use the most and fill smaller containers for easy use. Stick to the smaller containers for those used less frequently.

Keeping spices in larger containers helps to retain flavor due to larger containers not being opened frequently. Place in smaller containers for everyday use. Many spices have great health benefits, but some can be a problem (and potentially dangerous) if used in large amounts. Check your medications and make sure you understand which spices could have a negative interaction. Large amounts of nutmeg with certain drugs can be deadly. Spices contain what is in the soil and rain, just like all food items. That includes poisons and heavy metals, which can be found in brand name or organic products. Poisons and metals build up in the body and are difficult to get rid of. Countries like China and Vietnam have less safety rules than our FDA. Just because the label says grown in the USA does not mean it is. Herbs used in supplements can often contain, in part or whole, soybean, wheat and rice.

Meat.

Animal meat should spring back when lightly pushed in with a finger. If it is mushy and does not feel firm or spring back, it is old. It should not stink or have a gamey odor. Fish and seafood should not have an odor and be evenly colored. If there is any green, it is not safe. It should be bright with no dark spots and have a metallic shade to the skin or shell. The meat should be soft, tender and firm. Prawns and scallops may be a bit soft, but also firm. Learn how to choose quality meats and always check the date. Avoid products in ready-made sauces and breading because those can cover up aging meats. Stores and restaurants won't throw things away if they can sell them in different ways.

Beef in the grocery stores can be pumped full of dye to give a healthy appearance. Beef and bison should be grass-fed and deep in color. Avoid beef, like filet minion, that has been formed by putting pieces together. The mystery glue that's used for this is just that—a mystery.

Avoid lunchmeats and similar items. You have no idea what is really in them. Most contain nitrates and high amounts of gelatin and salt. Some canned meats, such as tuna and salmon, can be handy. Fake tuna will look much whiter than real tuna. Who knows what else is being used. Fresh is always better, but convenience is also important. Do what you need to and know where to draw the line. Canned ground meat is likely very high in sodium and not something I would usually choose to purchase.

Ham is a controversial meat. I sometimes buy a small bone-in ham and slow-cook it with pineapple or pear juice, spices and a little brown sugar. I then freeze portions in baggies for sandwiches and fried ham with eggs. Meats retain their nutrients for about three months in the freezer, then quickly lose them. Meats are like all animal foods: the quality is based on what they are fed.

Vegetables.

Root vegetables such as onions, potatoes and carrots should be free of blemishes, soft spots and dark areas under the skins. Garlic is difficult because most comes from China and can be bleached to look fresh. Look for garlic that still has part of the stem on it, as China cuts this off for easier shipping. Ginger is so delicious when fresh. Choose one the same way you choose other root vegetables. Green onions and asparagus can often go bad quickly. Plan to use these types of vegetables as soon as possible.

Yellow squash and zucchini can be lovely to eat raw or lightly sautéed. Acorn, butternut and other squashes are great, but they have a higher sugar content. They also can be a bit cheaper than other vegetables. Eggplant contains oxalates which contribute to kidney stones. It also contains cholinesterase, which blocks anti-inflammatory substances in the body. If you eat eggplant, do this on rare occasions.

Asparagus grows wild and can be found in many places. In character with lettuce, they are both easy to grow. Lettuce should not have a lot of moisture unless it's bib lettuce with attached roots. Prepare lettuce by washing it and letting it dry a little. Place a paper towel in its container to help keep moisture to a minimum. For spring-type mixtures in plastic containers, remove all moisture and place a paper towel above and below. This will keep it fresh longer.

Head lettuce has little to no nutrition. It is mainly water and fiber. When I eat salad fixings, I want the biggest nutritional bang possible. This means dark colors instead of lighter ones. *(Refer to the section on goitrogen enzymes.)*

Wash your vegetables! There are often insects and unwanted things on them from the fields and machinery. A black spider once came out of a celery bunch when I pulled off a stalk—after being in the refrigerator for a week! When it comes to celery and carrots, I wash, slice and store them in a container with a little water. This keeps them crunchy and juicy.

Most vegetables have wonderful benefits. Chinese vegetables are very good and sprouted beans are delicious. The best rule is to have a large variety, eating one root-type for every three above-ground types. Limit starchy vegetables such as potatoes. Watch what you put on them. Piling on a big blob of butter defeats the health benefits and covers up its flavor. As with all things, moderation and variety are the keys.

Sea vegetables.

These can be very delicious, but they're usually an acquired taste. These are very popular in Asia, and they have many uses for them. They can be nutrient rich. I believe they are worth a bit of research. Lack of exposure to these is one detriment to living far inland.

Seafood and fish.

Often, fresh seafood is hard to come by. When purchasing fish, look for wild caught, not farm raised. Farm-raised fish typically contain many toxins which have run into the water from soil. Many farms near fish farms use (or have used) chemicals.

Fresh water fish has the same issues. They can contain extremely high levels of toxins. Unfortunately, the world has become so toxic that it simply cannot be avoided anywhere.

Steelhead (a cross between salmon and trout) and trout are mild, sweet and convenient. I enjoy cod, grouper and a well-prepared bass. You won't know what you like unless you try it. Vacations are excellent opportunities to try new items. Local approaches to healthy items may or may not be healthy.

The ocean has its own problems with the harmful flood of sewage, mercury and the dumping of chemicals and plastics. When fish are able to move about freely, they are healthier and can get away from some of those heavy toxins. Anything kept in close quarters is ripe for stress-related health issues. Fish are designed to consume natural foods. Farm-raised fish are fed commercial fish food.

Most people do not know what type of fish they are being served at restaurants or what type they're purchasing in the frozen food departments. Once covered in batter or sauces, it can be confusing unless you know the meat source. The fish meat flakes should match the size of the fish. Asian catfish, tilapia and other cheaper fish have been passed off as grouper.

Atlantic cod has been overfished and vulnerable to extinction. Alaskan cod is a better choice. Atlantic halibut, flounder and sole are considered some of the worst wasted fish from fishing companies. They also contain high levels of contaminants, as most all things do these days.

Tilapia is a fish often used in restaurants and sold in stores. It is not a healthy fish and contains an unhealthy balance of Omega-3 and -6 fatty acids. It is associated with many diseases and health concerns.

Wild-caught Alaskan salmon is easy to bake or broil with a little Old Bay seasoning and a freshly squeezed lemon. I make a tartar sauce with mayonnaise, relish and dried onions (even a bit of dill). It's not that healthy, but I rarely have it. There is no need to buy commercial sauces. Many can easily be made at home and taste much better.

Compared to all other proteins, fish are easy and quick to make. They are also full of healthy oils.

Crustaceans.

Shrimp and lobsters have shells and are often referred to as crustaceans. Shrimp is easy to deal with, whether fresh or frozen. Be sure to get them deveined if you don't do it yourself. It won't hurt you to eat this, but the vein that runs along the back and tail is full of poop. Yuck. Try sautéing, steaming, baking, broiling and grilling to alter the flavors and change things up.

Crab is very rich and filling. It should be consumed in smaller quantities than most. It is delicious in dips, but these often contain unhealthy ingredients like mayonnaise. Shellfish contains selenium, which is necessary for the body's antioxidant defense system in preventing damage to cells and tissues. Crab is especially high in selenium.

Cocktail sauce is simply ketchup, horseradish sauce and fresh lemon. It's cheap to make and delicious. Fresh lemon goes with most fish, including crustaceans. It's healthy and lower in calories.

A lobster tail (preferably fresh, but frozen if you must) is low in calories, high in protein and delicious, especially when grilled. It does not need to be dunked in butter. A good lobster roll is an amazing and tasty meal on rare occasions.

Clams, mussels and oysters.

Eating these raw or undercooked can have huge risks. These are similar to crustaceans and are also considered shellfish.

Scallops are a great shellfish treat. A side salad with a scallop appetizer makes an excellent meal.

Some seafood and shellfish can be huge issues for people with health issues such as gout. Handling, storage and eating them raw can pose risks. Research this so you can make informed decisions.

Don't get in a rut with nutrition. YouTube and online classes are great for expanding your foodie knowledge and senses. Let your body tell you what it likes and does not like. I enjoy sashimi, but only maguro tuna. I once had food poisoning from a very nice restaurant with this limited choice. I will still eat it, but not very often. I'm even more careful about the quality of a restaurant where I make this choice, but that is still not a guarantee.

Life is full of risks, so don't get overly focused and freaked out. If you don't want something, don't eat it. You choose what goes into your mouth. However, there are times you should eat what is served so as not to appear rude. Use wisdom and be prepared by researching before such times.

Sauces.

I do not shy away from small quantities of heavy sauces. Heavy creams with the right herbs and ingredients are incredible. Dining out for these is a real treat since I don't usually have these types of ingredients on hand. French cuisine is one of my favorites. They really know how to make sauces and serve smaller portions. These sauces contain a good amount of fat and are very filling.

Many places have great signature sauces; however, many also contain a lot of sugar and a few unhealthy ingredients.

Sauces are often high in calories. General Tso sauce (a favorite) is not even a real Asian sauce, but became one anyway. It's tasty and has very high amounts of sugar. Know what is in them so you can make informed choices.

Tin foil, plastic and more.

Tin foil is made of aluminum, which you should avoid. If you use it, always place the shiny side toward the food. The dull side will flake off bits of aluminum into the food. This is also true for pots and pans and similar aluminum kitchen items. There are better choices. Get rid of pots and pans that are flaked and damaged.

All plastic items leach chemicals into whatever it is holding. The body can handle a good amount, but it can reach a tipping point for excessive toxins. The liver and kidneys could become overwhelmed. Plastics are a major part of life, but limit their use when possible. Glass is still a great option for storing items. Closed containers also protect from bugs and moisture. Many storage and carry options are available.

Use biodegradable and less toxic products in the kitchen, home and laundry. Become knowledgeable so you can make healthier choices. All this can seem overwhelming. Do what you are willing to and go to the next step when ready. My stainless-steel refrigerator door is not as shiny and fingerprint-free as others cleaned by chemical-based toxic products. I care more about my health and less about a perfectly mirrored finish.

The no-waste approach.

People waste too much. There are many ways to save time and avoid waste. If you tend to buy more than you need, adjust your buying habits and use the freezer for leftovers. The same meal can be altered as a later one after it has been frozen. There are basics to food preparation, cooking and storage; but they are not absolute. If you know about foods and how they are stored, you may feel comfortable extending the shelf life. If not, it is best to stay on the safe side. There is nothing that doesn't go bad over time, especially if it was not properly prepared and stored.

The FDA recommends keeping the refrigerator temperature below 40° F; I keep mine between 33°-34° F. The freezer should be kept at 0 F.

Never leave out foods of any kind. Put them away immediately after use. Allow hot items to cool a bit before placing them into the refrigerator. If placing in the freezer, cool in the fridge before moving to the freezer. Hot items can alter the inside temperatures of the refrigerator and freezer.

Condiments will retain flavor and last longer when put away immediately. This is a good habit which helps you remember. After defrosting (microwave, etc.), don't leave fish or chicken at room temperature for long. It is better to defrost gradually in the refrigerator. If you must defrost faster, use timers that remind you to check on it.

Check out the FDA storage basics and get familiar with the safety precautions.[20] They also cover how to handle the loss of electricity and non-refrigerated items. Don't guess.

Keep a list of what is in your freezer and label everything.

---

20 US Food & Drug Administration, "Are You Storing Food Safely?", February 9 2021, https://www.fda.gov/consumers/consumer-updates/are-you-storing-food-safely#:~:text=Keep%20the%20refrigerator%20temperature%20at,temperatures%20and%20are%20generally%20inexpensive.

Keeping certain staples around that you frequently use is a great idea, but buying too many perishables is very wasteful.

Make a game out of using up what you have. If you quickly or often go through something unhealthy like sugar, flour or mayonnaise, then cut back.

It's great to make things from scratch, but this can have a down side. For example, I noticed the organic, raw sugar in my pantry was going a bit fast. I had been making fruit jam (no pectin) and indulging in a bit of homemade caramel. I immediately made a correction by not making those items anymore. From time to time, our food intake should be adjusted.

Make a game out of not going to the grocery store. See how long you can go without restocking. This is a great way to force yourself to look further in the back of a cabinet, the freezer and refrigerator. Having extra of what you often use is a great way to plan ahead, but it is easy to forget things that get hidden and pushed to the side.

Get rid of the silly idea that leftovers are only for those less financially well off. Wasting is disrespectful and senseless. If you want to avoid leftovers, learn to make only what can be eaten at the meal. Save up the extra money for a wonderful vacation.

You don't have to eat everything in the name of not wasting it; just don't take so much. Put the utensils down (and the technology) and be present with your nutrition. Let go of attitudes that sabotage the respect and support for this vital sustenance.

Vacations.

Some people go on vacation and return 15-20 pounds heavier. Consider making it a game to come back a few pounds lighter. Choose from the healthy menus and skip desserts. You can have one amazing dessert, but not every night.

While on a cruise once, I was the only one at the large dinner table who ordered from the healthy menu. I made it a personal challenge to keep it up and refused to even look at the regular menu. It had nothing to do with the others, but I use them as an incentive to help me make healthier choices. One morning, I watched as a relative piled his plate high with about 20 pastries. He ate the whole thing! It made me feel sick, and it was an incentive to keep making healthy choices.

I did have a few unhealthy ones, but I kept them to a minimum and minded my body. I returned 2 pounds lighter and my relative came back 20 pounds heavier. He truly believed it was not a vacation unless he could stuff himself with *carboplunks.*

Take the time to learn about the staff and local traditions. It was an honor for an Indian waiter to serve me an extra piece of sashimi maguro tuna. We had previously chatted a moment about Ayurvedic views. In his country, an extra piece of protein is considered a great sign of respect. I did not want it, but ate it anyway. There are times to set aside one's desires to be kind to another. It may have been an insult otherwise. Caring about other beliefs, cultures and actions is compassionate and loving. This contradicts my choice of what goes in my mouth, but there are times to be adaptable and flexible.

Skin and hair.

There are very few legal requirements when it comes to cosmetics, skin care and hair care products. The packaging, labeling and list of ingredients all indicate nothing that would cause harm. If your shampoo or conditioner, for example, contains any of the following ingredients, it could be contributing to hair loss:

Sodium Lauryl Sulfate	Propylparaben
Sodium Chloride	Diethanolamine
Polyethylene Glycol	Triethanolamine
Quaternium-15	Phenoxyethanol
Methylparaben	Dimethicone
Alcohol	Propylene Glycol
Lanolin	Cocamidopropyl Betaine
Petroleum	Triclosan
Mineral Oil	Artificial Colors and Fragrances
Vitamin A	

You must do your research. This is why people often choose more organic and natural products that avoid such ingredients. Even then, you must research and ask questions. If people keep buying, there is no reason for companies to change ingredients. These types of companies care more about your dollar than your health.

There are many reasons to see a professional to help get you set up in the proper skin and hair care. Using aloe can be drying if not mixed with an oil, and mineral oil can burn the skin if not mixed with other ingredients.

Everything on and around you has toxins. Even healthy items like herbs, teas, healthy mixes and essential oils have side effects that can be harmful. The best way to avoid this is to research the side effects or hire a professional. It took a lot of research for me to make the smoothies I mentioned earlier. Most anything can have adverse reactions with medications. Make sure to read the warnings on all medications. If you question anything, ask the pharmacists, who are all trained in this.

Invest in a book about toxins in and around the home. In 1985, I bought a wonderful book that changed my life. Did you know that a popular baby shampoo, which gives the impression that it is mild and does not irritate the eyes, contains a numbing agent to keep the eyes from stinging? Whatever goes on the body gets into the body.

Try this: Rub a piece of garlic on the bottom of your feet. Within two minutes, you will taste it in your mouth. That's how long it takes to go through every capillary in your body to reach the mouth. This should also clue you into removing shoes when entering your home after being in areas treated with chemicals.

I use a little coconut oil in my hair mask and sometimes in my body oil. There are more calories in these products than people think when it comes to properly designing them for hair and skin. Many alternative professionals (myself included) will personalize recipes for clients. Individualized recipes can be made over and over, and with proper use can help the skin to overcome environmental challenges, feel more comfortable and look lovely. I designed a skin oil recipe just for this book in the Recipe section. I hope you love it as much as I do.

Making soap is pretty easy these days. Many kits offer a base, and all you need to do is add essential oils and other ingredients that fit your needs. Make sure the person designing soaps and similar products has the background to do them correctly. Homemade soaps don't usually lather up as much as commercial soaps, but they are cleansing and moisturizing. You will also need to package it so it can store without losing nutrients. There is nothing wrong with buying a quality organic soap made by others, even if commercially produced.

Shampoo and conditioners are a bit trickier. One must experiment to find the right ones. It helps to have two different kinds so you can use them interchangeably to re-stimulate the body. People living in very cold, hot and dry climates can have issues with hair flying away. This can be very annoying and uncomfortable. I mix two conditioners to help keep this from happening. Once, my hair was so crazy that I rubbed a dryer sheet (chemical-free, of course) on it to eliminate the static. If you must use a commercial conditioner to help with fly-aways, use on the lower part of your hair and avoid the scalp.

After some unexpected hair loss, I wanted to know why it was happening. I discovered my hair products contained every ingredient known for hair loss. Natural products can be slow to take effect. They require much patience and consistency. After a year, my hair started to slowly and steadily fill in. It may take a couple more years, but that's okay. I want healthy, long-lasting results, not up-front results that don't last. These types of products can take a while to get used to because they are oil based. Some may be too oily or not enough. It all depends on your climate and hair. The wave and shine in my hair have returned. It is not oily, brushes out easily, and the absence of split ends tells me that my body approves.

I have been highly pleased with a specific organic skin care line over the past many years. Making everything is very time-consuming. There are many quality organic makeup choices available. I want to put forth my best appearance; makeup can pop out my better features. We are human in a world of expectations. Do what you can.

Health starts from the inside out. Start where you are and do what you can. There is no better feeling than rising above the smoke and mirrors to be, feel and live your best!

8| Connection

It is most important to have a quality human experience by connecting with the self, others and the world around us. This desire runs deep and can be difficult to obtain in a world full of contradictions, controls, misrepresentations and obscurity. The world wants to tell you whom to trust, what to believe, and to avoid real connection. People are far less controllable and influenced when they have connections that are honest, supportive and reliable. Going through life without anyone to bounce ideas off and share experiences is tragic. When people are deeply connected with themselves and others, they have the necessary guidance and support to make better decisions and avoid painful and costly pitfalls.

People experience divisiveness from birth. We are divided over belief systems, culture, location, skin color, age, gender, and so on. Division creates an imbalance in the culture. If unchecked, the environment will tend to support those who would exploit this imbalance. For example, instances of bullying have increased over the last few years, especially in elementary schools. If a child is perceived as inferior (an imbalance), a bully may exert power over him. This action stems from false ego and a shallow sense of superiority. Bullying happens at every level in society.

In some circles, people speak of how emotions and feelings are not real and that we should ignore them. All emotions are created because of the thinking behind them. If the thinking is off, so will be the emotions connected to it. Feelings are Divine communications that provide guidance and assistance.

As a child or adult, maybe you experienced a moment when you thought emotions and feelings were worthless. *Toughen up. Don't be a big baby. Don't ask questions.* Without a connection to feelings and emotions, these powerful Divine communicators cannot guide and direct as they are meant to. And if we don't ask questions, it's impossible to learn and develop. These dividing concepts are the easiest way to create disconnection. They create unhealthy fears and insecurities, and only serve to separate and sacrifice healthy and necessary self-love. We must first have self-love to fully love another.

Post Traumatic Stress Disorder (PTSD) is at epidemic proportions. Serious complex PTSD often comes from horrific war or extreme cult experiences. Wars are politically and corporately motivated and are centered on control and profit with little to no respect for the damage it causes to people's lives. It is archaic and disappointing that the world should be damaged and destroyed by such savage approaches. Many other opportunistic scenarios result in similar endings.

In PTSD, the brain reacts to protect itself and the body

from harm. If an experience, thought or alteration intensely counters deeply accepted beliefs or is beyond the brain's capacity to comprehend, the physical body (including the brain) can react in devastating ways such as a heart attack or psychoactive event.

The brain steps in to protect itself and the one it serves, which is you. It shuts down whatever it doesn't need in order to not overload itself. Your body is 90% energy. As with electricity, it can overload when the wires cannot handle the amount of current. This creates excess heat and melts the cord, which sparks and catches fire, thereby destroying itself. If not caught early, it can reach beyond itself, creating further destruction.

The thought of war causes a deep emotional reaction in me. I went to elementary school outside an Air Force base where servicemen and women were sent for issues like alcoholism, drug addiction, in-home violence and the like. There had been two murders across from my home and there were apartments with little red lights that let people know prostitutes were available there.

I grew up with these people's kids. My best friend in third grade was already a speed drug addict, and I began carrying a knife for protection. Many of us grew up in difficult and violent homes. We were tough. Physical fighting was common. If you cheated at tetherball with me, lied to get me in trouble or bullied me, we would be meeting after school.

This was during the Vietnam war. Every student in that school would freeze and go silent when the principle's footsteps were heard coming down the hall. We would all turn and look at the window in the classroom door to see if she was stopping here. When she peered through the window, our hearts would drop into our stomachs. We focused on her face. If it was white as can be, we knew. The classroom teacher would go to the door with her face equally as pale. She'd walk over to the student who had lost someone they loved and cared about. The teacher would help the student gather up his/her things, then shuffle together over to the principal.

Two to three days later, the child would be thrown back into school unable to handle it, but was later granted leave to grieve for a couple of weeks. Being an empath, I felt everything from everyone. It happened over and over. I can't hold back my tears of compassion and sadness for such suffering. It was and still is devastating. Nothing has changed; now children have to worry about being shot in their schools. There is a loss of trust, frustration, helplessness, being insignificant, invisible and so much more. It is symptomatic of PTSD.

In order to be raised healthy, children need caring and attentive adults to develop healthy social and emotional intelligence so they can learn how to manage stressful moments and resolve issues into positive experiences. This empowers children and deepens their ability to connect with themselves and others.

Most parents who did not come from such positive environments are unable to provide such an atmosphere for the healthy development of children. Expressing authentic emotions of sadness, fear and anger are generally frowned upon and sometimes punished. Children often learn to abandon or stifle themselves for the sake of tending to the needs of others (PTSD fawning response; a component of complex PTSD). They serve and cater to those around them in order to please and not cause any issues.

As an extreme example, a doting parent, authority figure or institution may place a child on an undeserving pedestal. The child imagines he/she is the center of attention and can simply rule others. A child may ultimately decide his/her own needs supersede those of others, which can result in narcissism and selfishness. There are also parents who isolate the other parent to ensure dependency from a child throughout adulthood.

All these scenarios cause deep insecurities, harsh self-criticism, self-loathing and self-harming behaviors. It creates co-dependency, depression, pain and illness. These can lead to additional behaviors like alcohol abuse, defensiveness, dishonesty, food abuse, drug abuse, sexual abuse and other damaging thinking and behaviors.

If you are one of the lucky few who was raised with healthy parent figures, be aware that external factors can create similar damage. For example, a healthy person may end up in a situation where she feels trapped, unsafe with no way out, is emotionally and/or physically abused and is being controlled under fear of violence. This can precipitate not only PTSD fawning, but also PTSD freeze. With PTSD freeze, a person simply cannot move. They don't want to do anything because in that moment they feel safe. It's as if a heavy energy were laying on top of the person. She then beats herself up because she knows she has things to do and cannot move. It is an awful experience that easily supports depression and feelings of hopelessness.

It can be very confusing when anger, insecurities, rage or fear rise up with no apparent rational reason. It causes embarrassment, the desire to control others or situations, defensiveness and a whole slew of self-doubting and damaging emotions, behaviors and thoughts. This quickly expands and affects everything and everyone around. It may even create PTSD in others who are nearby and exposed to it. They never know if someone will be set off or if they can rely on a person to follow through.

There are many other forms of PTSD which are barely noticeable to a person, much less a professional.

I swear I have computer PTSD. My brain gets wired to expect something to happen (because it often does), which disrupts getting something done smoothly. When we expect a result, this sets energy in motion, and it becomes highly likely it will happen. If you golf, have you ever thought about not hitting the sand trap? What tends to happen? Exactly what you did *not* want. Instead of just noticing the sand trap, you probably thought: *Don't hit the sand trap!* You put your focus on it rather than the shot. Focus is in the moment and does not allow space for anything other than what you observe. Keep your expectations on the goals. The sand trap *just is*, and nothing more.

Consider a time when you ignored something you really needed to get done, but it was overwhelming and you couldn't bring yourself to even begin. It felt unmanageable because of its many parts, but it needed to be broken down into smaller and more manageable parts. The desire to ignore the uncomfortable feelings is strong. It must be overridden in order to take that first step, which can make the situation more manageable.

You may have looked at someone and could not figure out why they think the way they do. Let's use hoarders as an example. Over time, hoarders have rewired their brains to bypass any emotions they do not want to face. To them, they are thinking just fine. They learn to avoid the truth, burying it deeper and deeper. Their eyes no longer see and their noses no longer smell. Climbing over stuff becomes the norm for them. Parting with their items is not possible because it would mean a loss of control or protection.

Unhealthy thinking has attached false connections with the items where excess equals love, success or whatever else fills the void to keep them in this lifestyle. They ignore their embarrassment and compensate by no longer having visitors because they try to hide it from others. Their thinking is created by others and past experiences, and is also influenced by the world. Their chemically-altered brains bypass any notion of having reached a horrible condition that threatens safety and health. It becomes so ingrained and overwhelming that they are unlikely or unable to recover without help.

Hoarders' brains are wired to support their strong beliefs. The world is aware of this brain phenomenon. It is used as a means of dividing and stagnating human growth. If you deeply believe something, nothing will change your position, even when truth slaps you in the face.

Science has proven that certain foods and ways of thinking are sabotaging. Change is not disrespectful to beliefs. Conversely, beliefs are disrespectful to the process of evolution. Beliefs are meant to evolve into new awarenesses and truths. You are meant to change your views as you grow and receive more knowledge. The brain was meant to continue learning and changing so that the mind, body and spirit can do the same.

You did not get here by yourself. You have had much help. Consider noticing where your thinking is not serving you. As you begin to notice, more instances will come up. This is how you broaden your thinking. Just because science (or medicine) says so, it does not mean it is true. It should be a consideration, but not the only one. Training the brain to never change goes against the soul's design for change.

Consider how advertising and media add to this. They are riddled with unhealthy behaviors and violence. They compare us, our relationships and our lives to a fake worldview and set standards which are simply not real. As you watch over and over, your brain gets rewired to one view. You have probably asked someone a question and gotten an answer to a completely different question. Maybe the conversation went in a completely different direction. That person had most likely predetermined beforehand your responses and theirs. They were prepared to have a conversation based solely on their way of thinking. That person was not in the moment at all and certainly wasn't interested in an outcome different than theirs.

It is fine to prepare and have answers to expected questions, but to think a discussion will happen only one way is dismissive of anything that does not fit. Be present with what is happening in the moment. Adjust your thinking when it does not go the way you expected.

Let go of the past, embrace this moment, be honest and

start where you are right now. You are meant to know this stuff and to take a closer look at your healing and health. Learn how to build a life that lessens fear and stress in order to attract pure joy and happiness. You cannot change the world, but you can focus on what you can change—yourself, your thinking and your relationships. Remove the energetic garbage and replace it with healthy energetic nutrition. Do the work, take classes, listen to people who uplift, and share in a manner that brings about new awareness. The body and mind will step up to the emotional and physical plate you feed it every time.

Don't make food such a time-consuming focus. Too much attention on eating is unnecessary. In fact, eating simply is very easy. There is little cleanup if you eat an apple, peel an orange or throw together a simple salad. Healthy eating is a part of self-care, but it's not the only focus. Listen to what the body is telling you and act accordingly. In this amazing life, there are many talents to develop and beautiful things to discover about yourself and others. Keep learning and keep doing. Movement is necessary for the mind, body and spirit.

Miracles happen when you stop complicating things with overthinking. Read, sing, dance, walk, breathe, meditate, pray, explore and be open to that which is unfamiliar. In other words, *live*. It makes life exciting and fulfilling. It opens the pathway to learning and reconnecting with yourself and the world. We learn how to love in the midst of diversity.

There will always be challenges. There are no guarantees. However, if you take these ideas and move forward with more empowerment, you will be more prepared to handle things with greater ease.

Be honest with yourself and others. Lying is draining and stressful, and it only creates a fake self. Just because people don't always speak up does not mean they do not have thoughts. Too often, people think they are fooling others when they really aren't. Don't live in lies and pretense. In fact, telling the truth is a huge key to development. It is meant to be hard sometimes because it stretches you and gets you out of your safe box.

An introvert may be tempted to lie in order to move away from the conversation or situation. This is a missed opportunity for growth. There is always a way to say something kindly. Lying only confirms the belief that you are not capable of doing something any other way. This could keep an amazing opportunity at bay. Have the wisdom to know when to keep your mouth shut. You choose how your brain is wired.

There are times when a person may lie because of what is going on. If someone told me under threat of death to say the sky is purple, when it is in fact gray, I will say the sky is purple. Use common sense. However, realize that if this behavior is done many times, it can and will rewire the brain.

Quality of character and life experience is far more beautiful than youthful or perceived perfect appearances. The real you is incredible, big, beautiful and so amazing. You only need to look within to discover it. You have so many qualities that have been buried and forgotten; bring them to the surface. To help remind you, try a numerology or intuitive reading, psychotherapy or a hypnotherapy session. There are many alternative choices out there.

Advertising and powerfully influential media are based on the brain-wiring concept. I once had a person show me how to put toothpaste on my toothbrush. He was convinced I was doing it wrong. He methodically showed me how to curve and loop the paste to make two full layers on the brush, just like the TV commercial. It was silly, wasteful and ridiculous to me. I just continued with what has worked for me. There are many ways to accomplish the same thing. One way may or may not be better than another.

Thinking there is only one way makes it impossible to learn new things. Be open to new ways of doing and thinking. Every human has this issue because the brain is such a belief-supported system.

Beliefs will evolve as you learn more and more. Children do not start their education at the high school level and expect to understand much of anything. We must start nearer to the beginning, conceptually, with smaller ideas so we can develop an understanding of ideas and steps before moving on to bigger and more complex ones. Even steadfast beliefs will change as human education moves forward.

The efforts to control the majority of humanity are ongoing. Anything that influences how you think has a bit of truth and non-truth. You are meant to grow beyond what you believe from the past, present and future. The powers that rule the world know all of this. They fully understand how easy it is to wire the brain with repetition and strong experiences. People can become firm believers in something even if it makes no apparent sense at all.

People justify being members of cults despite witnessing the torturing and suffering of others. Some believe that if you do good elsewhere it can make up for damage and cruelty you either witnessed or participated in. Others defend belief systems shrouded in devilry and evil so long as they personally decide not to join in on their atrocities. Cults are powerful and have a major impact on this world.

There are many famous people in the Illuminati, for example. Many support and idolize these individuals. Some even publicly admit it. Even writers of famous books have endorsed scripts handed to them by this group. The Illuminati (enlightened ones) are one of several powerful secret societies. They are involved in the foundation of belief systems, culture and government. Their teachings are believed to incorporate Egyptian hermetism, Christian Gnosticism, Jewish kabbala, alchemy and other occult beliefs and practices. Their history is believed to have begun around the second century during gnostic times.

These types of secret societies hold certain universal knowledge the rest of us are not allowed to know. Great efforts have been (and remain) in place to keep those secrets to this day. They underlie and influence everything.

I once watched a televised interview with a gorgeous woman actor as the guest. She told the interviewer that she was male and had male parts. He laughed and laughed. She repeated this statement even as the interviewer continued to deny it and brush it off. He was obviously attracted to her but his thinking would not allow him to accept the truth. It was right in front of his face and he still denied it. His brain was just not open-minded enough to accept what he was being told. Living in denial was easier than entering the uncharted and uncomfortable waters where that interview could have gone. It was a huge missed opportunity for a powerful interview.

Everything you do and think affects how the brain supports you. Nothing is immune to this. It is also the same with addictions. Being a bitch, a grump, demanding, unreliable, driving aggressively, struggling with passing a fast-food place or believing in the need to eat tons of food are examples. If you can understand this concept, you can take over your own thinking. This is a game-changer!

If you've ever played a game where you did not understand the rules, you were likely at a disadvantage. You are in the game of Earth life, and the majority are at a disadvantage because of it. This is why secret society schools exist—to keep the majority from knowing the rules and all the players. Even their students get a manipulated version; otherwise, it could weaken control from those who rule and influence events. Humans are not, nor have they ever been, the only beings here. There is much hidden to keep control of the game. It has always been this way.

Put some thought into this, but not fear. You are here because you are capable and ready to figure this out. You are ready to move humanity forward. Our species is amazing and has much to offer this Universe, but it cannot be accomplished until you take over your own thinking and learn how to master it.

One of the biggest factors in the game is that you have psychic and intuitive skills. Every human is a sixth sensory being. You may not have all the skills, but you have some.

Regaining these requires some help. There are many who teach the development of these skills, from opening the mind's eye (for knowing) to understanding Divine communications in feelings and emotions. It is vast and incredible, but quality knowledge is important. Even in alternative approaches, individuals can get stuck in limiting beliefs.

I have heard teachers claim that all you need to do is trust the first thought that comes to you. There is more to this if you wish to have accuracy. Just saying you are psychic does not make you a developed one. Your personal views will influence accuracy if you are not aware of how and when to deal with them. There is much to learn before it becomes natural. This is true in most things.

One of the best skills is the ability to channel, which allows other life forms here and beyond to speak through you. There is no need for them to enter your body, but there is a need to connect. A quality channeler can connect with the past, present and future.

Learning from proper and quality teachers is an eye-opening education. There are many great channelers and skilled hypnotherapists who can help you channel. There is a belief that you cannot put yourself into hypnosis for such things, but I guarantee that is not true. I do it all the time. There are natural limitations and rules that must be followed. For example, you will not discover winning lottery numbers.

My favorite hypnotherapist and channeling colleagues are Alba Weinman and Pamela Aaralyn. You do not have to agree with it all, but consider it to get you thinking beyond your own limited earthly experience. Let go of the belief that intuitive or psychic individuals are not to be trusted. Those in control want you to believe that you cannot access such guidance and to ignore anyone else who can. This is not true. Those who channel can provide some amazingly accurate details and information that will speak to your soul. Choose that which resonates with you. Let your spirit be your guide.

If you find yourself rolling your eyes and getting impatient, this specific information may not be for you. Your soul may be directing you to a different type of session. Allow yourself time to put thought into it. This opens up a whole new level of earthly and Universal understandings.

Divine communication abilities and skills take time to develop. Most younger people are highly psychic, but have no idea how to deal with it. The quality of your character plays a big role in your connections and staying on the positive side of things. Evil people have these skills, but not the ability to tap into the positive and freer side of things.

As a person advances, so must the skills and knowledge. You can make yourself vulnerable to the negative if you do not learn how to avoid and handle such things.

The spirit within this Universe is aware of what is happening everywhere at all levels of life. It has a broader and deeper level of knowledge and information. There are also positives and negatives. There are some places you should never try to go.

Once, in a hypnotherapy session, I wanted my client and myself to meet her unique guardian. I was told spiritually not to go there. It would have blown her mind and obviously was not my place. Sylvia Browne once told me that curiosity kills the cat, It is true, and I heeded the advice.

The Universe is a very supportive system without negative or positive bias. I define negative as having control and decision-making over people, as well as imposing an overall lack of freedom for creativity and growth, individually and collectively. The positive (light) side supports freedom for all so each can soar to great heights. When spirit is allowed to guide and advise, the roadmap becomes clearer—sometimes shocking—and you move forward more quickly. Sometimes it holds you back because the time is not yet right.

The energetic and physical brains have a process for teaching that builds on what was taught and learned before. This is why we tend to move on when we come across something that does not feel right or is beyond our scope. The goal is to work with this knowledge in a way that does not push on a pull door, so to speak. Allow yourself to be guided. Stop watching television and start watching channeling (the spiritual kind). It is healthier and feeds the mind.

Consider listening to Russell Targ, an American physicist. His videos are on YouTube and other places. He speaks about how physicists tap into the knowledge in the energetic field (spirit) and are now proving how remote viewing occurs. Governments and corporations no longer hire psychics; they hire physicists for such things. It has been proven that science and spirit are connected and cannot be separated. They support each other. What is known today will evolve into a higher and different understanding in the future.

Connecting with feelings is highly important to Spirit's ability to communicate. Plants, trees, rocks, animals, dirt, earth and the atmosphere all communicate energetically through feelings. Emotions are based on thinking that has been molded through your experiences and choices. Feelings are soft, gentle, bold or severe communications from the field of information. They can guide, protect and clarify; and most of all, they have a shift that can be felt. This can lead to more profound and deeper understandings.

The Divine is the energy of life, the first life that began here in the Universe. There is no separation. All life and all things are connected to it. It provides the information you can use to better yourself and your life. This is why people do meditation and learn to clear all thought, letting go of distractions and tuning into whatever feelings are present. Animals do this all the time. They feel, then think, then act. They are so sensitive that they perceive the feelings of the atmosphere, energy/spirit and the physical.

A mountain goat cannot jump across one cliff to the next if it stands there and thinks about it. Athletes know this. They train through repetition (cell memory) so they can let go of all distractions and be connected through feeling with little thought beyond the basic accuracy of their performance and staying alert to avoid injury. They cannot depend on just where they are. If they are capable and wish to continue competing, they must gain new athletic and performance skills.

Life is a competition with yourself. When you learn, you discover new things related to your unique life experience and knowledge thus far. This information can be added into the knowledge in the energetic field, which in turn can likely help someone else.

Most small children have their psychic connections still intact. They naturally know, remember, and can access information. As they grow, these connections diminish very quickly. By four years of age, they have learned through societal trappings that these connections are not acceptable.

When an intuitive sensation occurs, it can happen in many ways. Information or words can seem out of context with what is going on. It is often very soft, gentle and subtle. One may even be reminded of an experience that can help better understand what is going on. This can cause people to question and doubt.

Sometimes, people can be on autopilot or maybe utter something totally unexpected. When I held my eldest son for the first time, my fantasy was looking into his eyes and lovingly welcoming him to the world. Instead, I blurted out, "Oh, I will have to watch you for appendicitis!" At 10 years old, he started having those symptoms. When I pushed on his appendix, he curled up in a ball of pain. I suggested a diagnosis and arranged for a surgeon on my own. This upset his new pediatrician greatly. His situation was life-threatening, as his appendix had seeped poison all over the intestines and body cavity. He needed a highly skilled surgeon.

It was not the first time I fought for one of my children's health. I do not recommend such actions unless you have knowledge and skill to support it. It was appropriate for me and the situation. Any quality mother knows that if something threatens the children, the ego disappears and the mama bear comes out. Nothing else matters beyond getting your children the proper help they need.

As you remove blockages in your thinking, you open up new awarenesses about yourself. This is how you discover yourself—the excellent, good, mediocre, bad and the ugly.

You must discover them in order to resolve them. Entrepreneurs get caught up in this one. Developing a business, parenting and being in relationships often force healing to the surface, which must be overcome in order to have success. Growth continues to occur at all levels as you venture into deeper levels of understanding. You can take better care of yourself with much less resistance. Learning never stops. That is who you are.

I am sharing with you not to convince, but to help you understand how this works. I believe understanding can be influential and make life easier within Universal rules. Considering another view can bring new perception within your life experience. Connection requires sharing, consideration, accepting diversity, connecting and defining communications, resolving emotional communications, and embracing the love of learning and change.

You learn even when you fail. Reject the stigma of failing; it is only a label. Those who fail over and over are refusing to give up. Conversely, they may not be learning or making the right decisions, so patterns will keep repeating until they figure it out.

When you find yourself stuck in a pattern, examine it from a different angle beyond the thinking that got you there. Choose differently so you can get around it, because repeating it becomes more costly. Don't do it all on your own. You can streamline the process by getting whatever help you need to solve the problem.

There is a duality in the idea that positives have opposing negatives, with each force emanating from a central point toward its opposite direction. This is differentiated by light and shadow aspects within the Jungian archetypes. We are our biggest blockage. Acknowledge it, learn about it and take action to correct it.

When you recognize your own vibration, you become aware of the connected and nearby vibrations of energy. Properly define them and they will communicate more clearly as time goes on. Spirit shares more if listened to, just like you share more if you are listened to.

To feel your vibration (your energy), you must clear out thinking and have presence with yourself. It always boils down to giving yourself permission, believing that you can and just letting go. Think of jumping on a trampoline. You have faith because you have done it before (experience). You trust in feeling the energy in the atmosphere as you land (energetic). You now have a physical connection (sensation) with the trampoline. This is energetic nutrition. It gives clarity, understanding and guidance to what you learn so you can move forward. This process moves you up the universal educational ladder.

Think about how the brain wires itself and where you might be stuck or influenced in ways that do not serve your best interest. Do what you need in order to safely and lovingly heal the brain. Heal any gaps with feelings, emotions and physical impulses of energy. You have a say in all this.

This book has shown an approach to physical and energetic nutrition. The world must go in a different direction, so learn how to play the game. Consider the mind's power to serve and to change just for you. When people realize they have the ability to alter and influence their own minds and tap into Universal communication, human wisdom can return in full force.

Emotions make us aware of what really underlies our thinking. This world is full of insecurities and self-doubt. This leads to miscommunications, misinterpretations and divisions, which lead to more insecurities. When you tune into this, it will lead to more *a-ha* moments for you.

Epiphanies are powerful. They create new awarenesses that bring deeper understandings about yourself and the world around you. This is the road to wisdom, and it can only be achieved with experience. Wisdom is the nourishment needed for any species to grow. It cannot be learned alone; we need the Divine and each other. Healthy and deep connections are what our souls crave most.

Through channeling, I have asked if there are any other reasons why we come here. The answer was:

> *You are here to have a sense of physical experience like that of taste, to feel a sense of separation* [Everything energetic is connected and there is no real separation. You are an individual, but also connected with the collective.] *and to grow and evolve the physical brain. You are to gain knowledge of how to better participate and live in eternal life with self and the collective purpose. Most of all, you are here to get through difficulty and return to a simplicity based in love. You are experiencing for the Divine* [all that is beyond us], *yourself and for others. You are meant to lose yourself, then rediscover yourself.*

Love is the key and is always at the foundation of everything positive. Be love.

You must learn to love and deeply know yourself so you can truly and properly love others. You can reboot your thinking and actions with more accuracy and greater ease. You can help the world change and thrive in the midst of chaos.

The changes you make may be unsettling if you have been stuck in the old you. Some people will be happy for you; others may feel the need to move on. Some may even try to pull you back to the familiar person you used to be. It can be hard for others to see you change, so be kind. Change is rarely easy or comfortable, the past fights for its place, but only what was learned can move forward with you. The rest must be left behind.

Mega-corporations are taking over the food chain and eliminating local farmers and ranches, and ultimately anyone who is not a part of their financial support system. More fake and unhealthy food will continue to grow. It is up to you to take steps for yourself to feel and be healthy and vibrant. Stop allowing these corporations to shape your views of nutrition. Start finding unhealthy items unappealing. Your valuable life and health depend on this.

The ongoing and increasing expense of maintaining lifelong health through medicine can be life-shattering. Much pain can be avoided by supporting your incredible body with the nutrition it requires. If it is not directly from unaltered nature, then drastically reduce (or avoid) consuming it.

As you reboot, reclaim and refocus nutrition at all levels, your health, life and relationships will change for the better—and so will the world. The more you embrace this type of living and *be-ing*, the greater impact it will have on world. Earth is waiting for us to step up.

Tap into a higher level of accurate guidance. You are capable of knowing and recognizing truth for yourself. You can remove the power of negative influences and take some of the difficulty out of life. Your healthier experiences will allow you to refocus on the more joyful parts of your life. Make the world a more fascinating and interesting place. You will then invite miracles and reclaim that childlike excitement and wonderment for living.

Nutrition Pyramid

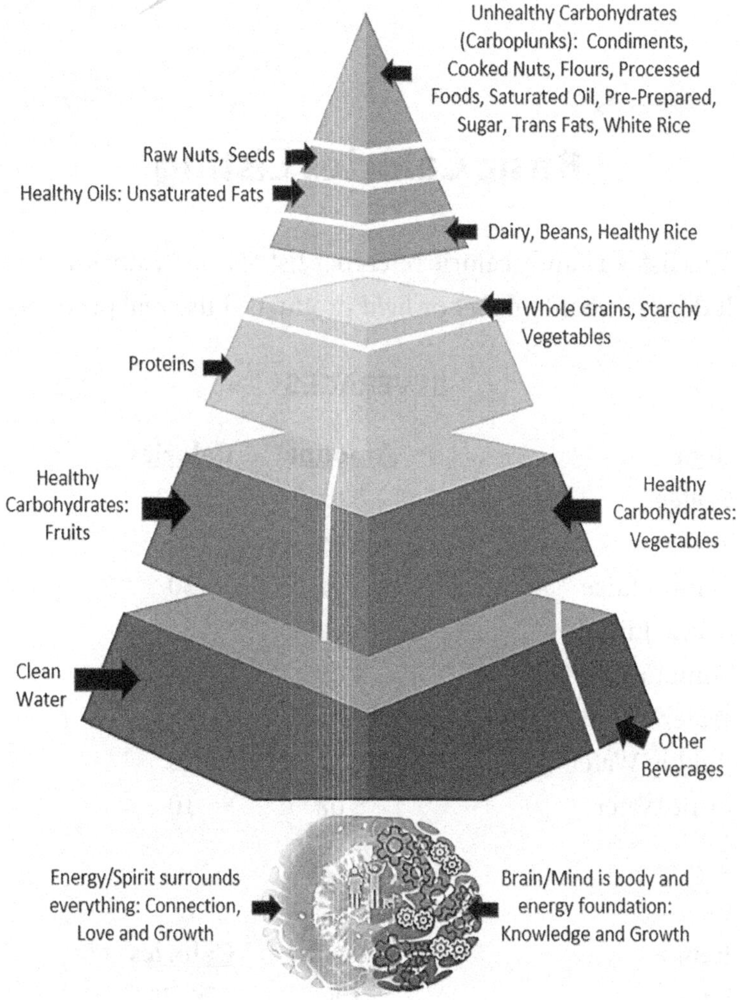

Basic Calories Listing

This list is a handy calorie reference list of lower calorie foods. It does not contain *diet* or *light* products. I use real products.

BEVERAGES

Item	Amount	Calories
Coffee	8 oz	0-12
Tea	8 oz	-2
Lemon Juice	4 oz	30
Prune Juice	4 oz	21
Tomato Juice	4 oz	25
Water	8 oz	0
Bubbly Water	8 oz	20
Fruit Water	8 oz	10

ENTREES

Item	Amount	Calories
Eggs	1 lg	74-78
Egg Whites, raw	1 lg	17

Item	Amount	Calories
Fish:		
White Fish	4 oz	81-109 *(cod, bass, mahi-mahi, flounder, grouper haddock, perch, snapper)*
Trout, Salmon	4 oz	108-153 *(mullet, salmon, scallops, shark, tuna, whitefish)*
Halibut	4 oz	158-240 *(herring, mackerel, milk fish, salmon-sockeye)*

Item	Amount	Calories
Meat:		
Alligator	3 oz	197
Beef:		
Bottom Round	3 oz	139
Brisket Flat	3 oz	174
Chuck Roast	3 oz	179
Ground Beef	3 oz	215
Beef Cotto Salami	1 oz	58
Eye Round	3 oz	138
Broiled Flank Steak	3 oz	158
Filet Mignon	3 oz	179
80% Ground Beef	3 oz	230
Rib Roast	3 oz	131
Rib Steak	3 oz	81
Roast	3 oz	169
Roast Beef Lunch Meat	1 oz	30-35
Salami	1 oz	73
Salami, lean sliced	1 oz	45
Short Ribs	3 oz	65

Item	Amount	Calories
Sirloin Steak	3 oz	236
Top Sirloin Steak	3 oz	166
Stew Meat	3 oz	201
T-Bone Steak	3 oz	177
Tenderloin	3 oz	168
Top Round	3 oz	177
Bison:		
Ground	3 oz	202
Roast	3 oz	123
Chicken:		
Spicy Buffalo Wings	3 oz	261
Breast, skinless	3 oz	128
Sliced Breast	oz	67
Drumstick/Thigh	3 oz	149-174
Liver Paté	1 oz	57
Lunch meat	1 oz	30
Duck:		
Breast	3 oz	119
Duck, roasted	3 oz	238-287
Lamb:		
Loin, Ribs, Sirloin	3 oz	160-183
Ground	3 oz	241
Other Meat:		
Emu Filet/Ground	3 oz	259
Goat	3 oz	122

Item	Amount	Calories
Pork:		
Bacon	.2 oz	34
Canadian Bacon	1 oz	42
Chitlins	1 oz	66
Chop	2.6 oz	149
Sirloin	2.5 oz	142
Ground	3 oz	253
Hot Dog	2.7 oz	204
Prosciutto, slice	.5 oz	50
Pulled w/Sauce	3 oz	147
Ribs	3 oz	199
Roast Center	3 oz	169
Quail:		
Whole	3 oz	199
Sausage	1 oz	120
Scrapple	.5 oz	44
Tenderloin Roast	3 oz	139
Veal:		
Breast	3 oz	226
Cube Steak	3 oz	220
Ground 8%	3 oz	146
Leg, cubed	3 oz	160
Top Round Steak	3 oz	128
Loin Chop	3 oz	185-192
Loin Cutlet	3 oz	242
Shank Roast	3 oz	151
Short Rib	3 oz	143

Item	Amount	Calories
Shoulder Steak	3 oz	168-171
Sirloin	3 4 oz	121-127
Turkey:		
Breast	3 oz	161
Dark Meat	3 oz	159-188
Giblets	1 oz	315
Gizzard	1 oz	139
Ground 11% Sausage	3 oz	146
Heart	1 each	34eart
Leg Roast w/skin	3 oz	177
Neck, skinless	1 each	243
Jerky	1 oz	71-81
Venison:		
Chop	3 oz	177
Stewed	3 oz	145
Seafood:		
Crab	3 oz	83-177
Crayfish	1 each	70-74
Lobster	3 oz	83
Shrimp	3 oz	101

GENERAL

Item	Amount	Calories
Soup/Stew:		
Beef/Chicken Broth	1 cup	15-17
Soup (no carb)	1 cup	75-150
French Onion Soup	1 cup	369
Fowl/Noodle	1 cup	31

Item	Amount	Calories
Beef Stroganoff	1 cup	173
Beef Vegetable	1 cup	32
Chicken Vegetable	1 cup	70
Oyster Stew	1 cup	135
Vegetable Stew	1 cup	70
Beef/Chicken Stew	1 cup	40-78
Soup Broth	1 cup	75-150
Broth, Cream	1 cup	600-800
Vegetable Meat Soup	1 cup	28-143
Beef Vegetable	1 cup	32
Chowder:		
Chicken/Vegetable	1 cup	70
Lobster Bisque	1 cup	246
Mushroom	1 cup	96
Oyster Stew	1 cup	135
Vegetable	1 cup	70
Veg/Beef/Chicken	1 cup	50-78
Fruit:		
Apricot	1 each	17
Apple	1 each	72
Apple, Crab	½ cup	42
Applesauce, no sugar	1/3 cup	33
Avocado	¼ cup	58
Berries	1 cup	53-66
Blueberries	½ cup	41
Cherries	1 cup	31
Black Cherry	¼ cup	44
Sour Cherry	½ cup	37-44
Dried Cherry	.5 oz	60

Item	Amount	Calories	
Clementine	1 each	40	
Dried Coconut	2 teaspoon	55	
Cranberries	1 cup	44	
Dried Cranberry	2 Tablespoon	45	
Currants	½ cup	31-55	
Dates	1 each	22-23	
Elderberries	¼ cup	26	
Fig	1 md	37	
Grapefruit	½ md	41-60	
Kiwi	1 md	46	
Kumquat	3 oz	60	
Lemon	1 each	15	
Lime	1 each	20	
Nectarine	1 md	70	
Orange		1 md	70
Papaya	1 sm	59	
Peach	1 md	38	
Pear	½ md	50-59	
Pineapple	½ cup	37	
Plantain chips	.5 oz	74	
Plum	1 md	30	
Prunes	3 md	50	
Rhubarb	1 cup	26	
Starfruit	1 cup	33	
Tangelo/Mandarin	1 md	45-50	
Tangerine	1 md	45-50	

Vegetables:

Alfalfa Sprouts	½ cup	5
Artichoke Hearts	½ cup	58

Item	Amount	Calories
Asparagus	5 oz	25
Bamboo, cooked	5 oz	17
Beet Greens	1 cup	8
Broccoli Flower	1 cup	32
Broccoli	1 cup	44
Brussels Sprouts	1 cup	38
Cabbage	1/8 head	27
Carrots	½ cup	27
Cauliflower	1 cup	34
Celery	1 cup	17
Cherry Tomato	1 cup	27
Collard Greens	1 cup	49
Cucumber	1 cup	16
Eggplant	1 cup	35
Endive	½ head	44
Green Beans	1 cup	38
Cooked Kale	1 cup	36
Lettuce	5" or 1 cup	21
Mung Bean Sprouts	½ cup	16
Mushrooms	4-5 each	15
Mustard Greens	1 cup	15
Onion	1 sm	29
Peas, raw	½ cup	13
Peas, cooked	½ cup	35
Peppers	1 each	12-18
Bell Peppers	1 md	30
Radish	½ cup	7-15
Sauerkraut End	1 cup	30

Item	Amount	Calories
Seaweed Kelp	½ cup	18
Snap Beans	1 cup	27
Spinach, raw	1 cup	11
Spinach, cooked	1 cup	41
Squash	1 cup	25-38
Squash, Summer	1 md	31
Swiss Chard, cooked	1 cup	35
Tomato	1 md	18-35
Tomato Pastes	1 Tablespoon	13
Turnip, cubed	1 cup	36
Zucchini	1 md	35

Grains, Starches, Nuts & Seeds:

Almond, raw	1 Tablespoon	62
Barley	1 Tablespoon	50
Brazil	1 each	32
Buckwheat, cooked	¼ cup	160
Bulgar Wheat	¼ cup	160
Cashew, raw	1 Tablespoon	50
Coconut	1 teaspoon	18
Farro	¼ cup	200
Flax Seeds	1 teaspoon	45
Freekeh	¼ cup	160
Mullet, puffed	1 serving	85
Oats	¼ cup	152
Pecan, raw	1 Tablespoon	45
Walnut, raw	1 Tablespoon	45
Wheat	.5 oz	52
Wild Rice	¼ cup	160

Item	Amount	Calories
Dairy:		
Cottage Cheese	¼ cup	58
Condiments:		
Au Jus	2 Tablespoon	5
BBQ Sauce, low sugar	1 Tablespoon	5 (low sugar)
Capers, drained	1 Tablespoon	2
Creole	¼ cup	25
Curry	1 Tablespoon	9
Horseradish	1 Tablespoon	7
Ketchup	1 Tablespoon	15-17
Marinara	1 Tablespoon	9
Mayo	1 Tablespoon	100
Mayo Light	1 Tablespoon	46-50
Mole Verde	1 Tablespoon	15
Mustard	1 Tablespoon	10
Oyster Sauce	1 Tablespoon	5
Black Olives	5 lg	25
Green Olives	5 each	50
Picante	1 Tablespoon	4
Soy Sauce	1 Tablespoon	11
Steak Sauce	1 Tablespoon	5
Taco, red/green	1 Tablespoon	5-7
Tahini	1 Tablespoon	85
Tamari	1 Tablespoon	10
Vinegar/Balsamic	1 Tablespoon	5-12
Wasabi	1 Tablespoon	2
Worcestershire	1 Tablespoon	11

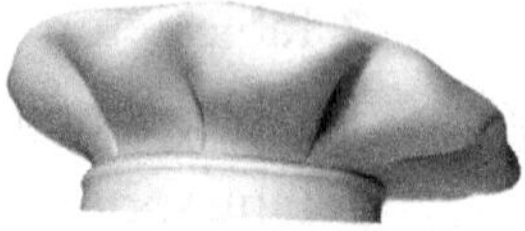

Recipes

Here are a few of my favorite recipes that are simple, mostly healthy and tasty. There are many ways to substitute, so feel free to look for options. I hope you enjoy these.

Hummus

Makes 2-¼ cups. 2 Tablespoons equal about 55 calories.

- 4 cups water
- 1-1/2 cups dried chickpeas
- 1/2 teaspoon baking soda (aids in tenderizing the beans for smoother results)

Gently simmer the above on the stove, covered, for 2-½ to 3-½ hours (check occasionally), or save time and use an appropriate instant-type pot, until tender and easy to smash. Drain a cup of the liquid into a heat resistant measuring cup. Drain the rest off the beans. Place beans in a food processor and add:

- 1/2 cup of the bean liquid (save ½ in case you need to add a bit more)

2 tablespoons sesame tahini
2 tablespoons fresh Lemon Juice
1 teaspoon garlic powder
1-1/4 teaspoons sea salt
1 teaspoon ground cumin

Blend in processor until light, fluffy and smooth for about 3 to 4 minutes. Slowly add more water if too thick. Store in tightly covered container in refrigerator for no more than 2 weeks.

Serving ideas: Serve at room temperature or slightly warm, drizzle a bit of good olive oil (about 120 calories per tablespoon) on top or a drizzle of reduced balsamic vinegar. Can serve plain, with pitta bread, crackers, bagel, chips, clean raw or slightly cooked vegetables (celery, carrot, mild bell peppers, lettuces, zucchini), top with toasted pine nuts, grilled and spiced chicken and as a side to a salad.

Hummus is very filling. Be careful not to eat too much.

Dressings, Marinades and Sauces (store in refrigerator for about 2 weeks):

Apple Cider Vinaigrette

1/2 cup apple cider
3 tablespoon apple cider vinegar
1/4 Granny Smith apple, peeled, cubed
1/2 teaspoon salt
Dash teaspoon ground white pepper
3/4 cup grape seed or olive oil

1/2 tablespoon minced tarragon
1 teaspoon pure maple syrup

In small saucepan, simmer the cider until it is reduced by half. Add vinegar, apple, salt and pepper in a bowl. Gradually whisk in oil. Stir in the tarragon, maple syrup, and adjust seasonings as needed.

Serve immediately or refrigerate for later.

Balsamic Dressing

1/2 cup olive oil
1/4 cup balsamic vinegar
2-3 teaspoon honey
1 teaspoon dijon mustard
1 shallot (or green onion greens) minced
1 clove garlic, minced or 1 teaspoon garlic powder
1/8 teaspoon onion powder
salt and pepper to taste

Mix all ingredients.

Blue Cheese Dressing

1 cup mayonnaise
1 cup sour cream
3/4 cup buttermilk
1 teaspoon crushed garlic or 1 teaspoon ground garlic
1/2 teaspoon dry mustard
1/2 teaspoon salt
1/2 teaspoon sugar
1 pinch cayenne pepper

1 teaspoon Worcestershire sauce

4 ounces crumbled or grated blue cheese

Mix all ingredients carefully, folding in any crumbled blue cheese. Cover and place in refrigerator for at least 3 hours or overnight.

Citrus Vinaigrette

1 Orange

1 Lemon

1 Lime

1-1/2 Tablespoons Honey

1 Tablespoon Champagne Vinegar or White Wine Vinegar

1 teaspoon Sea Salt or to taste

1/8 teaspoons black Pepper

3/4 cup extra Virgin Olive Oil

Use a rasp-style grater to zest the peel of the orange and lemon. Squeeze half the fruit juice to make 2/3 cup. Place into bowl and whisk in honey and vinegar. Slowly drizzle in olive oil and vigorously whisk or blend.

Greek Lemon Dressing

1/4 cup fresh lemon Juice

1-2 teaspoon dried oregano

1 large garlic clove minced

1/4 teaspoon sea salt

1/4 teaspoon black Pepper

3/4 cup extra virgin olive oil

Whisk lemon juice, oregano, garlic, salt and pepper in a bowl until combined. Slowly drizzle in the olive oil as you vigorously whisk.

Oriental Salad Dressing without Soy

2	tablespoons olive oil
1	teaspoon sesame seeds (lightly toasted, place in dry fry pan and heat to lightly brown)
2	teaspoons ground ginger
3	tablespoons pure maple syrup
1-1/2	tablespoon cider vinegar

Mix the above and enjoy on salad or a vegetable dip.

Honey Mustard Dressing

(1 cup)

1-1/4	teaspoon pure maple syrup
4	tablespoons honey
2	tablespoons whole grain mustard
1	tablespoon brown or dijon Mustard
1/4	cup apple cider vinegar
1/2	cup grape, avocado, or olive oil
2	crushed garlic cloves or 2 teaspoon ground garlic
1/4	teaspoon salt
1/4	teaspoon pepper

Wisk the above until smooth and to your taste. Mix before each use. May need to let rest a bit to warm up at room temperature.

For creamy honey mustard dressing, add 1/4 cup mayonnaise.

Hot Salad Topping Dressing

Sautée on medium any vegetables such as the following:

1 tablespoon avocado, grape seed or olive oil to sautée the following:

- onion (add a dash of sugar and sea salt to bring out flavor)
- yellow squash
- mushroom
- broccoli or any vegetable you have on hand.

Start the vegetables first. When lightly cooked, add a splash or two of Balsamic vinegar, stir and plop it all on top of salad leaves.

Strawberry Vinaigrette

2 strawberries for processor plus 1 sliced for garnishing the salad
1 tablespoon apple cider vinegar
1 tablespoon fresh lemon juice
sugar to taste
Dash salt and pepper
Dash cayenne pepper

Combine all ingredients in food processor. Purée until smooth. Pour over salad and garnish with sliced strawberry. Can use as a marinade or sauce for chicken.

Chicken and Salmon Marinade

1 tablespoon olive oil (optional)
1 whole fresh lemon juiced

2 crushed garlic cloves or garlic powder
2 fresh chicken breasts

Mix the above and place in baggie with chicken breast. Marinade overnight or place in freezer for another time. From frozen, defrost in refrigerator for 1-2 days.

Serve grilled, baked, broiled or sautéed.

Portobello Mushroom Marinade

2 Portobello mushroom caps placed in closable plastic bag

Mix the following and add to bag:

1/4 cup balsamic vinegar
1 tablespoon avocado, grape seed or olive oil
1/2 teaspoon garlic powder or crushed clove
1/2 teaspoon onion powder

Carefully remove the dark substance under mushroom cap. A grapefruit spoon with serrated edges makes this easy. Rinse and carefully dry off. Mushrooms can break easily. Place marinade and mushrooms in bag. Refrigerate overnight.

Grill on medium high heat and grease the grate for about 5 minutes. Broil 5-7 minutes.

Serve alone or as a hamburger patty substitute.

Apple Chicken Salad

3/4 cup chicken, diced
1 apple, diced
3 stalks celery, diced
3 tablespoons fresh lemon juice

1/8	teaspoon cinnamon
Dash	nutmeg
Dash	cardamom
•	salt to taste
•	honey, agave, maple or some type of healthy sweetener to taste

Mix ingredients together, drizzle with lemon juice, mix sweetener with cinnamon, nutmeg, and cardamom and drizzle on salad. Chill a minimum of 20 minutes.

Serve with chopped walnuts or raw almonds. Can mix in a low sugar Greek yogurt or 1 tablespoon mayonnaise for a creamier texture.

Cocktail Sauce

2	tablespoons ketchup
1/2	teaspoon horseradish sauce
•	fresh lemon juice to taste

Mix the above and enjoy.

Great with cooked shrimp

Store in a tight container in the refrigerator for no more than 2 weeks.

Mango Habanero BBQ Sauce

Fabulous Wing Sauce!

1/2	diced onion
1	deseeded diced habanero pepper
1/2	mango, diced (optional)
1	tablespoon oil

1 12-ounce can crushed tomato
2 tablespoons tapioca flour or corn starch
1/3 cup soy sauce
1/3 cup molasses
1 cup mango vinegar (easy to make, if store bought add a more diced mango)
1/4 cup brown sugar
2 tablespoons honey
1 teaspoon garlic powder
1/8 teaspoon smoked paprika
1 tablespoon pure maple syrup

Sautee onion, habanero pepper in oil until soft and a bit caramelized. Add diced mango, tomato, flour or starch, soy sauce, molasses, vinegar, and brown sugar. Simmer for 10 minutes.

Place in food processor and add honey, garlic powder, smoked paprika, and maple syrup. Blend until smooth.

Orange Chipotle Barbecue Sauce

1/4 cup chopped fresh cilantro
1/4 cup frozen concentrated orange juice
3 cups water
1-1/2 teaspoons crushed chipotle chili peppers (ground works fine)
1/2 cup canned diced tomatoes, in juice
1 teaspoon ground cumin
1-1/4 cups champagne vinegar
3/4 cup honey
3 tablespoons dijon mustard
6 cups cattleman's classic (or similar) barbecue sauce

In a large, heavy bottom sauce pan, combine all ingredients except barbecue sauce. Bring to a boil over high heat, reduce heat to medium and boil for exactly 30 minutes.

Remove from heat and strain mixture into an appropriate storage container. Add barbecue sauce and stir to combine mixture.

Store up to 7 days in refrigerator.

Serve with ribs or pulled pork.

SOUPS

Light and Healthy Mexican Soup

- 2 cups chicken bone broth, heated until very hot
- 1/4 teaspoon chicken soup base or sea salt to taste

In serving bowl add:

- 1/2 diced fresh avocado
- 1/2 diced medium fresh tomato
- 2 tablespoon diced green onion greens

Pour hot broth on top of vegetables.

Salmon Chowder

Small cooked salmon piece will equal 1/4 cup broken up.

- 1/2 cup chopped carrots
- 1/4 cup chopped celery
- 1/4 cup chopped onion
- 1/2 cup water
- 1/4 cup broken up cooked or canned salmon

1	cup milk
1/2	teaspoon butter
1/8	teaspoon garlic powder
•	salt and pepper to taste

Boil vegetables in water until tender. Add salmon and milk. Heat until very hot. Add seasonings to taste. Cook 1 minute, then add butter and serve.

Serve with toasted bread, or cut bread cubes to place in chowder (optional).

Tomato Soup

1	28-oz can whole tomato (blend in blender or processor until smooth)

Sautee the following:

1	tablespoon olive oil
1	medium diced onion
1	teaspoon ground garlic
1/8	teaspoon red pepper flakes (optional)
Dash	sugar
•	salt and pepper to taste

Add the vegetables to the smoothly blended tomato blend or process with vegetables. Add the following, as needed, to thin out:

1-1/2 to 2 cups chicken broth

Simmer in a pan for a few minutes before serving.

VEGETABLES

Avocado Tomato Salad (2 Servings)

- 2 tablespoons oil
- 2 tablespoons fresh chopped cilantro
- 1 tablespoon lime juice
- 1/2 teaspoon garlic
- 1/2 teaspoon dried oregano
- 1/4 teaspoon ground cumin

Mix the above well, then drizzle over the following:

- 2 medium tomatoes, sliced into wedges
- 2 avocados, peeled, and largely diced

Oven Roasted Vegetables

- asparagus, fresh and cut into 2" pieces
- red, yellow and orange bell peppers, roughly chopped
- red onion, roughly chopped
- zucchini, roughly chopped
- 2–3 cloves minced garlic
- 2 tablespoons olive oil
- salt and pepper to taste

Preheat oven to 450°. Place all the veggies on a baking sheet or a roasting pan. Combine in small container; garlic, olive oil, salt and pepper. Toss veggies with mixture and every 10 minutes while cooking.

Roast 20-40 minutes until tender.

Potatoes Au Gratin

2 cups diced ham (optional)
3 cups thinly sliced potatoes
2 tablespoons butter
2 tablespoons flour or tapioca flour
1/2 cup diced onion
1/2 teaspoon salt
1/2 teaspoon dry mustard
1/4 vegetable salt (optional)
1 cup milk
1 cup shredded cheddar cheese (optional)

Melt butter and mix in flour, mustard, salt, and milk. Microwave 3-5 minutes. Stir every minute until thickened.

Lightly oil an 8x8 baking pan. Layer with potato, onion and ham, and drizzle some sauce over it, repeat until covered. Bake in microwave for 15 minutes, or 375° oven for about 40 minutes. Test to make sure potatoes are tender. If microwaved, top with cheese when removed. If baking in oven, half way through cooking, top with cheddar cheese. Let stand 5 minutes before serving.

Roasted Bell Peppers

(5 servings)

2 pounds red and yellow peppers, cut into 1/4"-wide slices and drained in colander for 2 hours

Mix the following and add to drained peppers:

1/8 cup olive oil

1/8 cup raisins *(fun fact: sulfur dioxide is used to make golden raisins)*
1/8 cup pine nuts
1/8 cup chopped fresh parsley
1-1/4 teaspoons minced garlic

Serve immediately or refrigerate until ready.

Roasted Tomato

1-2 tomatoes, sliced, placed on cookie sheet
2 teaspoons olive oil, brush tops of tomatoes
• sprinkle of fresh thyme (or rosemary)
• sprinkle of sugar on top
• salt to taste

Bake at 250° for 2 hours. DO NOT open oven. Let sit overnight OR bake at 250° for 3 hours and serve immediately.

ENTREES

Beef Stroganoff (4 servings)

1/2 pound fresh mushrooms, sliced
1/4 cup onion, chopped
1 clove garlic, minced
1/4 cup butter, melted
1 pound boneless beef sirloin, cut into bite-sized 1-inch square or rectangle pieces
2 tablespoon all-purpose type flour
1-1/3 cup (10-1/2 ounces) chicken bone broth
3 tablespoons Burgundy (optional for beef Burgundy stroganoff)

1/4 teaspoon pepper
1 cup sour cream
• hot noodles, rice or toast

Sautée mushrooms, onion and garlic in butter until onion is tender. Add beef. Cook, stirring constantly, until browned. Stir in flour, broth, lemon juice, burgundy and pepper. Bring to a boil. Reduce heat and simmer gently for 15 minutes. Stir in sour cream and cook until thoroughly heated. Do not boil!

Healthy Chili

2-1/2 cups brown rice or whatever healthy grain you wish (cooked most the way in chicken broth)
2 tablespoons grape seed oil
1 quart fat-free, low sodium chicken broth
1 cup broccoli florets
3/4 red bell pepper
2 stalks celery, chopped (include the leafy tops for great flavor)
1 onion, chopped
1 chicken breast, cubed
3/4 cup pinto beans
2 tablespoons raw beet stalk tops, chopped
1/2 small can jalapeno, chopped, or 1-2 fresh jalapenos, chopped
1 small zucchini, chopped
1 small yellow squash, chopped
1/8 teaspoon red pepper flakes
1/4 teaspoon sea salt
1 teaspoon crushed garlic

1 14-ounce can diced tomatoes in juice
3/4 cup water
1-2 tablespoons chili powder
1/4 teaspoon sea salt
1/8 teaspoon Mexican spice (cumin, oregano, onion powder, garlic powder, ground chipotle or cayenne pepper, smoked paprika)

Heat oil in medium to large sauce pan. Add all vegetables, chicken, red pepper flakes and the ¼ teaspoon sea salt and sautée until lightly crisp. Mix all spices together and add to the sauce pan. Cook for 1 minute to bring out the spice flavors. Add water and tomatoes, chicken broth and brown rice. Cover and simmer for 1 ½ - 2 hours. If too thick, add more chicken broth.

Serve with shredded cheese like cheddar and/or a bit of sour cream.

Happy Chicken

(Serves 6)

4 chicken breasts, halved, boned and skinned (may use 6 chicken thighs instead)
• salt and pepper to taste
1 cup all-purpose type flour
2 tablespoons olive oil (or other high heat oil)
2 tablespoons butter
1 large onion, chopped
2 tablespoons freshly minced parsley (or 1 tablespoon dried)
1 16-ounce can tomato wedges or diced tomato

- 1/2 teaspoon ground cinnamon
- 1/4 cup packed light brown sugar
- 1 cup dry sherry or vermouth
- 1/2 cup raisins
- 1/2 cup slivered almonds or crushed walnuts

Mix flour, salt and pepper together. Heat oil and butter in skillet. Dredge chicken Flour mixture and cook in oil until browned. Place chicken in 3-quart casserole dish.

In same pan, cook onions until transparent. Add parsley, tomatoes with liquid, cinnamon, cloves, brown sugar, sherry, and raisins and simmer uncovered for 15-20 minutes, stirring occasionally. Pour over chicken and sprinkle nuts on top of mixture.

Bake uncovered at 375° for 30 minutes.

Halibut

- 1 pound halibut
- 1 lemon, zested, and juice
- 4 garlic cloves
- 1 tablespoon capers
- 1/4 cup fresh basil
- 2 tablespoons olive oil
- 1 teaspoon red pepper flakes (optional)
- • salt and pepper to taste
- • lemon slices for plates

Rinse and dry halibut. Mix zest, lemon juice, garlic, capers, basil, oil and pepper flakes. Brush on both sides of fish. Grill at 450° for 4 minutes each side.

Salmon

1-2 salmon steaks

- sprinkle with Old Bay seasoning
- fresh lemon slices

Rinse and dry salmon. Bake in the oven or a toaster oven, or on the stove in a pan with a touch of oil. Salmon should be medium rare for best flavor, moisture content and nutrition. Bake, skin side down, 400° for a total of 8 minutes; or broil for about 3 minutes. Weather affects cooking, and appliances do not all cook alike. Keep watch and note the recipe if the times are different.

Serve with fresh lemon slices. Salmon is very versatile. Add a drizzle of honey or maple syrup to change it up.

Grainy Salmon with Lime Topping

(Serves 2)

10 oz fresh salmon fillets
2 tablespoon grainy mustard
1/4 teaspoon lime zest
2 tablespoons fresh lime juice

Brush foil topped pan with a touch of oil. Turn on broiler and line a pan with foil (shiny side toward food), then brush with oil. Remove skin from salmon and place on the foil. Mix the zest (grated rind), juice and mustard. Spread on top of salmon. Broil 2 inches from heat. Measure the fish at its thickest point and broil 8-10 minutes per inch.

Lobster Tail

Frozen: Defrost and remove shell. Rinse and dry. Broil, grill or boil until done. White and pink. May spice with salt, garlic powder, paprika and onion powder. Can serve with fresh lemon. If desired, use melted, clarified butter (fat-free butter oil). These make a great side to a salad or sliced to top a salad.

Add a bit of mayo, diced celery, minced onion, paprika, mustard, salt and pepper for an amazing Lobster salad.

Steamed Shrimp

Clean shrimp by removing the head, peeling off the shell and legs, and removing the back vein (intestinal tract is fine to eat, but can have a bit of sand in it). Add flavor to the water in the bottom of the steam pan by adding a bit of wine, beer, fruit juices, broth, or whatever you like.

Add liquid to pot and any other seasonings you wish. Make sure there are 2 inches between bottom of pan and bottom of steamer. Make sure liquid is within ½ inch of the bottom of the steamer. Cover the pot and bring the liquid to boil over high heat. Reduce to medium and add shrimp. Replace cover.

Steam until the shrimp curl and turn bright pink. About 4-6 minutes for 1-2 pounds of shrimp. Shrimp should be firm to the touch but give just a little and have bright pink on it. Drop shrimp in cold water and keep refrigerated until ready to serve.

Barley Shrimp and Vegetables

1-1/2 cups chicken broth
1 teaspoon chicken soup base or bullion
3/4 cup barley (take out a tablespoon for topping)
1-2 stalks celery, diced
1 small onion, diced and sauteed
1/2 cup chopped broccoli tops, lightly cooked
2 tablespoons grape seed oil
1/4 cup diced cooked carrots
1-1/2 cups diced cooked shrimp
1/4 cup shredded parmesan
2 tablespoons pecans
1/4 cup additional shredded parmesan for topping

Simmer soup mix, broth and barley for 1 hour. Sautée onion, add broccoli and celery in oil. Mix all ingredients and top with Tablespoon of barley and ¼ cup cheese. Bake 375° for 20 minutes until bubbly and when cheese is melted.

Rinse off and dry all fish and meats. They will brown much better and it gets the packaging slime off of them. Learn about basic cooking. There is much available for every type and level.

All these recipes are adaptable. Find a substitute for any ingredient you wish. A bit of real and natural sweetener here and there is just fine. We are naturally drawn to sweet things such as in mothers' breast milk.

Fruit sugar is different than refined sugar. It is healthy, but in proper amounts. Honey, agave and maple are wonderful substitutes for sugar. Raw sugar is okay on occasion, but must be greatly limited when refined.

Keep things simple with an occasional complex item. Salad and baked vegetables are a wonderful meal. When you eat for nutrition, you will feel so good that your body won't want to go back.

Don't make cooking complicated. A simple salad of lettuce with a dressing, with baked onion, yam/or potato, bell pepper and other vegetables sprinkled with your favorite spices (garlic powder, onion powder, paprika, sea salt and pepper) are amazingly delicious and filling.

I hope these recipes give you great inspiration and maybe a new favorite or two. Recipes are all over the place, online and in books. Most everything can be made from scratch. The more self-sufficient you are with your food, the cheaper, more satisfying and healthier you will be.

Check out this bonus recipe below for natural skin care:

Body Skin Oil Recipe

(Makes approximately 16 ounces)

1-1/4 cups rosehip oil
2 tablespoons jojoba
1-1/2 tablespoon aloe vera fillet or gel or liquid (is also a preservative)
1-1/2 tablespoon vegetable glycerin
2 teaspoons castor oil
1 teaspoon vitamin E (is also a preservative)

For further healing and lightening of sun and age spots, add 1/2 teaspoon of pure frankincense or myrrh.

For very dry climates, dry skin or those with eczema, add 2 teaspoons lanolin (get one that is somewhat liquid). If your skin is rather rough add 1 tablespoon of snail mucus (I use this on my face before moisturizing).

Add the ingredients to your container. Shake well and before each use. After drying off from your shower or bath, apply the Body Skin solution. Top with your favorite lotion to help the oil soak in. Wait a few minutes before getting dressed. Keep the container on the counter until used up.

Keep all unused oil in the refrigerator and take out the night before so it can warm up and liquify.

Note: Keep in mind this is very oily. The container is likely to leak or leave an oil ring on the counter. I use a 16-ounce container with a heavy-duty medium sized pump. For traveling, always put your oil container (do not use a pump, as it is likely to leak) in a Zip-lock bag.

Always check with your pharmacist to make sure the ingredients do not affect other medications you may be taking.

Archetypes

Each person is made up of many archetypes. These are patterns in thoughts, feeling, images and behaviors that make up our personalities. There are well over 300 archetypes. The following is a partial list on some of the most common ones and their shadow effects. There are positive and negative aspects to each one.

In life, we experience both determinate and indeterminate events. If one of these archetypes hits close to home for you, take a close look at its shadow aspects. These can help clue you into parts of yourself that may need attention and/or adjustment. Examine the thinking and feelings behind those familiar to you.

WARNING: You are going to recognize your friends and family in these descriptions. Try not to correct or pass harsh judgement on anyone. Be a living example of growth and change, as this is always the best teacher.

Also take note of the talents and skills you may possess. Some may be hidden and some more obvious. Everyone is a mixture of these. Be honest and real, and don't beat yourself up. Keep growing and changing into the amazing person you are meant to be. If something does not fit, let it go.

Addict
recognizes when something has more authority over their willpower than does their inner spirit; creates a reference point when overcome; passionate

> *Shadow*: struggles with willpower and the absence of self-control; compromises integrity and honesty, relationships, finances and well-being; glutton; workaholic; gambler, stalker; substance abuse; conspicuous consumer

Extremely emotional and intellectual people struggle to balance these powers

Employment: likes regular hours, routines, reasonable working conditions that match commute needs and fitness abilities with clear expectations and room to grow; addiction counselors, teacher, therapist, physical health

Advocate
comes to the defense of others; champions their rights publicly; furthers social change; has a willingness to take action

> *Shadow*: has false or negative causes; commits to causes for personal gain

Employment: attorney, defender, legislator, lobbyist, environmentalist

Alchemist
converts some form of matter into altered expression of itself; spiritual development aligned to the laws of the universe; wizard; creative

> *Shadow*: misuses power and knowledge; brings seduction and trickery through magic.

Employment: wizard, magician, scientist, inventor, writer, artist, healer, psychologist, health & wellness, musician, research, yoga, dancer, psychic reader

Angel
dedicated to representing angels; artists; authors; has loving and nurturing qualities; godmother/godfather

> *Shadow*: making claims to be in touch with angelic guidance for the sake of control or ego; acting innocent or angelic to mislead others about their true nature; work/life imbalance

Employment: doctor, nurse, firefighter, emergency medical technician, lifeguard, social worker, teacher

Artist
passionately expresses a dimension of life just beyond the five senses; expresses animated psyche into physical form; chef, painter, landscaper; visionary; enterprising; entrepreneur

> *Shadow*: comprises many clichés; eccentric; genius; suppresses artistic talent for fear of recognition coming only after death; difficulty with structure

Employment: musician, author, dramatist, actor, artisan, craftsperson, sculptor, weaver, fashion designer, conductor, animal lawyer, film director, art director, actor, copywriter, talent director, singer, craft artist

Athlete

strength and human spirit involving code of ethics and morality; example of the universal power of the psyche; develops personal willpower and strength of spirit as a requirement for the body to manifest its perfection; includes handicaps; competitive; enjoys physical challenges; loves outdoors

> *Shadow*: misuses strength against any person or opponent; gamblers, bar fighters; lacks honor which compels them to cheat to win; extreme thrill seeking; focuses on weaknesses; overly competitive; sports focused; not living wisely, bully; fear vulnerability

Employment: Olympian, coach, nutrition, trainer, kinesiologist

Avenger

needs to balance the scales of justice, sometimes by aggression; volunteers for pro bono work; pursues corporations or war criminals; self-righteous on behalf of society on a global scale; guards against injustice to themselves or family; avenging angel suggests one is on a mission from God; leader, courageous; selfless, integrity; compassionate; uplifting

> *Shadow*: avenges immoral behavior by resorting to violence; has a burning desire to get even and may dedicate

a lifetime to that end; heavy focus on saving others; violence

Employment: film, television, drama, fiction, religion, pursuing businesses that damage society; justice; advocate

Beggar
is completely without material resources; depends on the kindness of others; begs for attention; loves authority and material objects; learns about the nature of generosity; compassion and self-esteem are fundamental to this archetypal pattern

Shadow: fanatic; martyr; saboteur; victim; harsh judging; entitled; aggressive; chronic begging; indigent; greedy; selfish; not giving back; in survival mode; outlaw

Employment: films, fiction, nonfiction, religion, fighter, soldier, fisherman

Bully
believes the spirit is stronger than the body; takes on bullies on behalf of others (like David and Goliath); heals wounds

Shadow: keeps others from discovering his true identity; coward; deep fears; anger; impulse issues; low empathy; easily picks out weakness in others; violence; revenge; rebel; passive/aggressive; wanna-be; relationship struggles

Employment: advocate, counselor, healer, video gaming

Caregiver

known as the "mother"; represents maturity and is ego-balanced; generous, protecting, loving, nurturing; unconditional love, compassion, dedication and patience; willingness to help others; puts other people's needs ahead of their own; easy to get along with; highly likeable; flexible; does whatever is needed; takes good care of self; brings order to chaos

> *Shadow*: can fall into Victim or Slave archetypes; spends too much energy on others; difficulty setting boundaries; often in basic survival both physically or emotionally; develops feelings of bitterness, anger, frustration and resentment; guilt-trips others; seeks recognition for good deeds

Employment: nurse, medical, psychologist, teacher, animal advocate/lawyer; nanny, art therapist, writer, music teacher/therapist, physician; clergy; career counselor

Child

courageous; artistic; fun; nurturing; works hard; spontaneous; magical; sense of wonder

> *Shadow*: needs approval; limiting; underdeveloped; wounded; brat

> **Orphan**
>
> reflective; tribal spirit; develops independence early; without family influences, attitudes, and traditions; inspired to construct an inner reality based on personal judgment and experience; life represents the fear of surviving

Shadow: never recovers from growing up outside family circle; feels abandoned and scared from family rejection which stifles maturity and may cause them to seek out surrogate family structures (therapeutic support groups who heal deep wounds); painful feelings of non-acceptance in the family

Wounded

holds memories of abuse, neglect and other childhood traumas; pain of abusive experiences; substantial influence on adult life; blames dysfunctional relationships; deep sense of compassion and desire to help other wounded children; spiritual perspective; very forgiving

Shadow: self-pity; tendency to blame parents for current shortcomings; resists moving on through forgiveness

Magical/Innocent

enchanted and enchanting to others; potential for sacred beauty in all things (horrific experiences, yet believing humanity is basically good); embodies qualities of wisdom and courage in the face of difficult circumstances; gifted with the power of imagination and the belief that everything is possible

Shadow: absence of the possibility of miracles and transformation from evil to good; attitudes of pessimism and depression, especially when exploring dreams; "once upon a time" dreams by cynical adults; belief that energy and action are not required, allowing one to retreat into fantasy

<u>Nature</u>
inspires deep, intimate bonding with natural forces; has a particular affinity for friendships with animals; has tender, emotional qualities; has an inner toughness and ability to survive; resilience of nature; develops advanced skills of communicating with animals; veterinarians and animal-rights activists have a conscious rapport with animals; feels they are communication with nature spirits and working in harmony with them to maintain natural order; must relate and care intimately for animals to the extent that the psyche and spirit need these bonds and are crucial for well-being

Shadow: tendency to abuse animals, people and the environment

<u>Puer/Puella Eternis (Eternal Boy/Girl)</u>
a determination to remain eternally young in body, mind and spirit; healthy attitude

Shadow: goes to extremes for appearance; double standards; avoids responsibility and may lie or exaggerate; may dress too youthful

Employment: jobs that help make the world safer, child advocate, healer, writer, teacher, counselor, special education

Clown

makes people laugh and cry; wears a mask to cover their real emotions; reflects the emotion of the crowd; represents what people would like to do or say themselves; great humor; motivating; a knack at stating the truth; good heart; wise; fosters living with kindness and simplicity like *Forest Gump*; humor associated with power and personal protection; enterprising; artistic; social; intelligent; talented

> *Shadow*: Clown or Fool manifests cruelly as personal mockery or betrayal—specifically, the breaking of confidences gained through knowledge from the inner circle; hides true feelings; likes attention; behavior grants immunity from retribution; feels undeserving; lacks realism; rebels against conventional; too agreeable; not conscientious

Employment: politics, stage/theater, film, comedian

Companion

takes care of day-to-day life details; service to a personality that often has a stronger nature or a role that carries more authority; associated with providing emotional (rather than sexual) support; anticipates needs of others; supportive friend and worker; easily switches roles; grateful; loyal; softens hard hearts

> *Shadow*: betrayal is common, which damages the soul; compares self to others such as others not being smart, pretty or better than they are; believes things would fall apart without them; stealing; servant; hoverer

Employment: community, service industry, working with animals, assistant, spiritual

Creator

willing to constantly be learning; ego is outward facing to the world; inner world is free of ego constraints; good at working out solutions; recognizes that connection with others is not only artistic but creatively supports both the physical and spiritual; constructive; ambitious; unique; does things with excellence; innovative; imaginative; expressive; visionary; accepts change; inspires

> *Shadow*: focuses on perfection; never completely finished; always wants more; not content with what they have; lacks stability and comfort; not in control of emotions, which creates chaos; struggles for connection in relationships; tends to exclude others from their lives; non-conforming; single-minded; perfectionist; stagnation; indifference; mediocrity; deep fears

Employment: stone cutter, piano tuner, jeweler, scientist, writer, inventor, art technology, marketing

Damsel

beautiful and vulnerable; similar to Princess, who is considerate of those around her and more often associated with romance than distress; sweet; aura of magic; also known as Maiden; self-sufficient

> *Shadow*: mistakenly teaches patriarchal views that women are weak and teaches them to be helpless and in need of protection; in need of rescue; demanding;

high-maintenance; feels powerless without a partner; yearns to be saved; drama; unhealable wounds; unfaithful; entitled; weak and powerless; disappointed expectations

Employment: fashion designer, makeup artist, hair stylist, party organizer, entertainment, dancer, costume dresser, writer, nurse, florist, wedding planner

Destroyer
destruction for reconstruction and rebirth; releasing that which is destroying us, such as emotion and behaviors; recognizes stages of rebuilding; resilient

Shadow: Destruction becomes an end in itself; generates death, madness and abuse; targets groups and/or individuals, nations, environment, relationships; promotes attitudes and opinions that destroy others' dreams or potential; criminal; immoral behavior; chaotic; tries to convince people that devastation can be controlled; suicidal; cruel; self-destructive

Employment: scientist, healer, therapist, relief and disaster, donations, causes that support rebuilding

Detective
ability to seek out knowledge and information; combines great powers of observation with highly evolved intuition to deduce solutions; inquisitive; enterprising; influencing; logical

Shadow: voyeurism; falsifying information; selling out

to the highest bidder; snoop; distrust; struggles with completing tasks in a timely manner; doubt; alienation; places blame without cause

Employment: spy, double agent, private investigator, profiler, warrior/crime fighter, leader

Don Juan
underlying vulnerability with its power to open a heart; capable of deep love: emotional independence; and the self-esteem to be immune to his manipulative skills; charming; confident; risk taker; sophisticated; sexually attentive; confident

Shadow: preys on women for conquest alone; falls into sex role clichés; radiates an attitude that all women need him far more than he needs them; invulnerable to women's charms; sex addict; manipulative; gigolo; Casanova; extreme risk taker; underlying fragility; makes a game out of seduction

Employment: party influencer, fashion, romantic type, travel careers, host, greeter, acting, modeling, advertising

Engineer
hands-on; devoted to making things work; reflects the character of grounded, orderly, strategic qualities of mind that convert creative energy into a practical expression; practical; strategic; considers others; advantageous; strives for solutions; spatial design, intuitive; highly creative

Shadow: ignores needs of others; master manipulator; seeks own advantage; selfish; money focused

Employment: architect, builder, inventor, costume design, make things work better, solving problems

Exorcist

pattern of exorcising negative spirits of others or of social groups or society; ability to confront evil in the form of possession by destructive or antisocial impulses in oneself and others; shaman; intuitive; willing to take on rigorous training and focus; neutralizes duality into oneness

Shadow: attacks evil in others without having the courage to face his own demons; invites darkness; addiction; mental illness; makes others feel wrong; lust over power; dark focus; imbalanced

Employment: clergy, psychologist, soldier/officer, psychic, medium, specialized shaman

Father

talent for creating or initiating the overseeing of others; courage and protectiveness; guides and shields those under his care; sacrifices own desires when appropriate; lifelong attachment to the role of family patriarch; oversees; leads; creates; compassionate

Shadow: Caring guidance and protection can turn into dictatorial control or abuse of authority; doctorial; tyrannical

Employment: leadership, creative designer, politics, real

estate, psychologist, therapist, counselor, teacher, writer, medicine, healer, clergy

Femme Fatale

female counterpart of Don Juan; reverses conventional sexual stereotypes; opens hearts of others; self-sufficient; enchanting; obtains many life skills; mysterious; glamorous; powerful; natural flirt

> *Shadow*: sexual and financial, whether from money and power inheritance or drawn to it; seduces men with money, power and survival; murderer; dominating; manipulative; emotional investing; manipulative; dependent; seductress; deceitful; conflicted with feelings; very flirtatious; lacks morals; self-gain

Employment: entertainment, spy, story teller, sales

Gambler

risk-taker who plays the odds; attempts to outrun the speed at which ordinary change happens; psychic; follows hunches and the belief in one's own intuition: willing to put in the hard psychic work needed to make relationships succeed; optimistic; logical; strategist; stamina

> *Shadow*: compulsive gambling, focused on finding ways to beat the odds; looks for lucky breaks in relationships; gut reactions; wasting time and effort toward a quick dollar; dreamer; energetic; intuition; schemes; willing to take dirty jobs

Employment: finance, detective, politics, real estate, statistics, stocks and bonds, insurance, sales

God

benevolent and compassionate; willing to use powers to help others out of love for humanity; lifelong sense of great power used unselfishly; heroic; generous; rules with kindness and love; strong leader

Shadow: easily becomes a dictator or despot, oppressing others with those same powers; uses physical attractiveness to get what they want; lifelong sense of great power used selfishly; dominating; power hungry; deceitful; disrespects life; desires worshiping; risking others; arrogance; power-hungry; deceitful; arrogant

Employment: CEO, human resources, politics, spy, medicine, legal, sports, environmental manager

Goddess

source of all life; fertility connection; inspires women, embodying wisdom, guidance, physical grace, athletic prowess and sensuality; lifelong associations with the image and personality associated with the goddess; wise; embraces spiritual traditions; beautiful; loving; heroine; strategist; intellectual; strong leader; creative; visionary; nurturing

Shadow: emerges from the exploration of feminine power, including the exploitation or overindulgence of movie stars and fashion models; self-image strongly connected with sexuality; over-indulgence; misuse of power; deceitful; arrogant

Employment: healing arts, spiritual arts, entertainment, politics, spy, speaker, writer, sales, counselor, science, military, useful crafts, aesthetic careers, medicine, legal, sports, healer, food industry

Gossip
connected to lessons of truth, integrity and honoring trust placed in them; confidant; confident; trustworthy; supportive; understanding; integrity; respectful; discerning; restraint; connections

> *Shadow*: spreads rumors, backbites and forwards exaggerated and harmful information intended to disempower; hounds celebrities; damaging rumors; misleading information; measures quality of relationships by whether a person shares secrets; uses information as currency; chaos; feels superior; riddled with underlying fears and insecurities; snoop; greedy; indifferent; irresponsible; power hungry; hypocrite

Employment: networker, private investigator, fraud investigator, digital photographer, police officer, gossip columnist, market researcher, personnel coordinator, client service associate

Guide
role of Teacher to a spiritual level; sees the Divine in everything; continuing pattern of devoting self to teaching others through own spiritual experiences; gains wisdom through self-disciplined practice, study and spiritual experiences; natural insight and acceptance of what is; rational and cre-

ative; does not waste words; spiritual mother; problem solver; calms chaos

Shadow: opportunistic televangelists and gurus of various traditions; more interested in financial gain; controlling; center of attention; know-it-alls

Employment: guru, sage, spiritual teacher, evangelist, healer, psychologist, psychic, medium, medicine

Healer
passion to serve others by repairing the body, mind and spirit; inspires others to release painful histories or make changes that redirect the course of their future; assists people in transforming their pain into a healing process; channels energy to generate physical or emotional changes

Shadow: takes advantage of those who need help; claims to heal any and every illness; exaggerates; money focused; narrow minded; wanna-be; gives too much to others; self-important

Employment: intuitive healer, caregiver, nurse, therapist, analyst, counselor, traditional and alternative medicine, jobs that serve others

<u>Wounded Healer</u>
initiated into the art of healing through some form of personal hardship such as non-curable illness or loss of possessions; trauma healing; pushes toward transformation rather than healing an illness.

Shadow: takes advantage of those who need help;

claims to heal any and every illness; unable to turn to others for support; deep fears; victim

Employment: same as Healer

Hedonist

seeks pleasurable aspects of life such as food, wine, sexuality and sensuality; healthfully self-indulgent; balanced; inspires creative energy to embrace good things in life; spiritual transformation; desire for the good life; mystic; lives in the present moment; spontaneous and flexible; optimistic

Shadow: pursues pleasure without regard for their own or others' health; self-indulgent; lacks balance; fear of being seduced and losing control in the physical world; manipulative; two-faced; achieves material luxuries at all costs; needs to succeed; fear of being captive or losing control; pursues pleasure at the expense of others and one's own well-being

Employment: sociable jobs, chef, gourmet, art collector, high end store, real-estate, mystical, design, fashion; sales

Hero/Heroine

capable of great feats of strength or skill; classic figure; confronts increasingly difficult obstacles in order in order to awaken man/womanhood; survivor; awakens inner knowing or spiritual power; desire to help others; unselfish

Shadow: can become empowered through disempowerment of others; manipulative; egoic; know-it-all; mental imbalances

Employment: waitress, actor, servant, assistant, military, politics, scientist, accountant, teacher, chemist, judge, medicine, veterinary

Judge

balances justice and compassion; manages fair distribution of power in any form; natural mediator and good with interventions; high standards related to justice and wisdom and the manner in which people interact; experiences aligned with forgiveness; lifelong learning process centered around justice and compassion

> *Shadow*: consistently destructive criticism; judging without compassion or with a hidden agenda; legal manipulation; misuse of legal authority; threatening others through an association with the law; misuse of business, legal and criminal authority; top dog over the little guy; negative; power hungry; restrictive

Employment: critic, examiner, mediator, arbitrator

King

an archetype of major proportions; the height of temporal male power and authority; utilizes and considers others' recommendations; keeps balance and harmony; wise; kind; mature

> *Shadow*: selfish rulership; tyrant, hypocrite or bully; driven to success; critical; power hungry; greedy; selfish; cruel; controlling; indulgent

Employment: positions of leadership, politics, attorney, sales, corporate design, government

Knight

primarily associated with chivalry, courtly romance, protection of the Princess, and going to battle only for honorable causes; self-sacrificing; spiritual overtones of service and devotion; loyal; great virtues; high standards; natural ability to get things done

> *Shadow*: absence of honor and chivalry; loyalty to a questionable ruler or principles; can fall into a pattern of saving others while ignoring one's own needs

Employment: inventor, mystic, diplomat, community protection, animal rights

Liberator

great military and political leader; frees tyrannical countries; liberates from self-inflicted negative thought patterns and beliefs; offers options to violence, suffering and spiritual stagnation; campaigns for freedom fighters; lifelong pattern of helping to free others from injustices, adverse economic or social conditions or from misconceptions; charismatic

> *Shadow*: can liberate from one tyrant only to impose their own tyranny over our lives (corporate, political, religious and spiritual); speaks of freedom as a way to individual aggrandizement; sluggishness; poor nutrition

Employment: military, politics, activist, psychologist, counselor, religious positions, economics

Lover

romantically inclined, great passion and devotion; lover of art, music, gardening, beauty; sense of unbridled affection and appreciation of someone or something; attentive; caring; love of family, friends and life; healthy emotion, feeling and idealism; lives in the moment; environmentally appreciative; passionate; forgiving; sensual; warm and inviting

> *Shadow*: exaggerated, obsessive passion causing a destructive effect on one's physical or mental health and self-esteem; high importance on physical appearance connected to self-esteem; fear being alone; self-sacrifice; luxury may outweigh common sense; lacks healthy self-love

Employment: caregiving, service industry, sales, entertainment, acting, writing, storytelling, music, activist

Martyr

knowingly or blindly represents a cause

> *Shadow*: utilizes a combination of service and suffering for others as the primary means of controlling and manipulating; self-sacrifice; manipulative

Employment: politics, religion, social work, activist, psychology

Mediator

smooths relations between potentially antagonistic groups or individuals; patient and skilled; reads people and situations with great acuity; sees and respects both sides; lifelong commitment to resolving disputes and bringing people together.

Shadow: ulterior motives or hidden agenda; works two sides of an issue for personal gain.

Employment: ambassador, diplomat, go-between, sales, human resource

Mentor

teacher in whom you can place implicit trust; passes on wisdom and refines that of others; concerned with aiding mind, body, and spirit; lifelong pattern of embracing individuals to guide many aspects of their lives; loves learning; exemplar of sharing and caring; respectful

Shadow: imposes control in lieu of wisdom; allows students to move into the role of master while maintaining control over their development of mind, body and skills; overbearing attitude

Employment: teacher, counselor, tutor, spiritual practice, business, master role

Messiah

embodiment of divine power and being sent on a mission by Heaven to save humanity; a sense of great purpose; kind; caring; loving; integrity; ethics; morals; enlightened

Shadow: obsessed with mission and spiritual purpose to the point of psychosis; hears voices directing him to take lethal action; subtle and difficult to identify; convinced that God needs them to do something bigger and better than others; egoic; loss of a sense of self; criminal

Employment: psychology, religion, activist, jobs that help others reach positions of leadership, teacher

Midas/Miser

entrepreneurial or creative ability; has the power to generate wealth for an entire kingdom; paramount in folklore; turns everything he touches to gold; generous with time and money; highly self-motivating; creative and innovative; strong sense of vision; confident; outgoing; optimistic; good at budgeting

Shadow: greed; hoarding; lacks generosity; a need to control surrounding forces for fear of losing wealth; difficulty maintaining relationships; selfish and demanding; perfectionist

Employment: professional positions, finance, statistics, accounting, investment, advertising, marketing, corporate finance and management

Monk/Nun

spiritual intensity, devotion, dedication, persistence and wisdom; extremely industrious and involved; single-minded, assiduous, devoted to a spiritual path or to any great achievement that requires intense focus; believes celibacy reserves energy for work and/or spiritual practice; worldly possessions and desires are not important

Shadow: religious recluse removed from the real world;

overly pious or privileged in being unconcerned about earning a living or raising a family; lacks connection

Employment: novelist, entrepreneur, service jobs, activist

Mother
life-giver; source of nurturing and nourishment; unconditional fountain of love, patience, devotion, caring and unselfish acts; keeper and protector of life from children to the family to the earth and all life; intimately connected to nurturing and protecting the environment; bond with Mother Nature is a lifelong devotion; wise; loving; caring; adaptable; flexible

Shadow: devours children psychologically and emotionally and instills feelings of guilt; abusive, abandoning, working mother (in crisis over being at home and working) representing different aspects within the community

Employment: teacher, counselor, psychologist, therapist, writer, story teller, careers with access to further learning, assistant, scheduling, project management

Mystic
extraordinary states of consciousness such as prolonged ecstatic trances and preternatural abilities of precognition or bilocation; spiritual: genuine enlightenment manifests as desire to be of service; cosmic explorer; intuitive state of mind; speaks poetically; attracts fans and followers; possesses unearthly wisdom; free spirit; ethical; high standards

Shadow: egocentric concern for one's own spiritual progress to the exclusion of others; an attendant sense of self-importance at having achieved higher states of consciousness; takes advantage of admirers or students in economic, emotional or sexual ways; spiritual seeker rather than a mystic; withdrawals from the world to live a solitary life; not grounded; grandstanding for money

Employment: health and wellness, teacher, psychology, counselor, homeopath, martial arts instructor, clergy, writer, musician, artist, alternative health, paranormal investigator

Networker

very ancient; expands sphere of influence by forging alliances and making connections among vastly different groups of people; military, social and clan alliances; helps develop social flexibility and empathy; helps others find empathy in order to find commonality with others; inspires groups; unites people; finds, draws and fosters connections; coordinates many possibilities

Shadow: uses others for personal gain; believes himself to be highly popular; tries too hard; overwhelmed by all the possibilities; takes over life; loses sight of goals

Employment: messenger, assistant, sales, marketing, journalist, writer, insurance

Pioneer

discovers and explores new lands, medicine or spiritual practices; initiates new fashions and arts; creates and does what has not been done before; needs to visit fresh and undiscovered territory; enthusiastic; intellectual inquisitiveness; gets out of comfort zone; risk taker; truth seeker

Shadow: compulsive need to abandon one's past and move on to the next conquest; does not consider getting lost or sticking to any schedule; involved in slavery; extreme risk taker dependent on adrenaline to feel alive; obsession

Employment: explorer, innovator, entrepreneur, agriculture, medicine, science, technology

Pirate
symbolizes freedom and the ability to strike at rich and aristocratic classes who gained wealth from labors of the poor; spiritual awareness in finding one's own value rather than pirating others' wealth; seeks freedom; energetic; driven

Shadow: steals both intellectually and informationally; acts of piracy, crime, or robbery; intimidation; likes to impress

Employment: treasure hunter, sailor, weapons, merchant, navy, escort service, bounty hunter, chef, landscaper, horse racing, farming, skip tracer

Poet
combines lyricism with sharp insight; finds essence of beauty and truth in affairs of humanity and in everyday acts and objects; great deeds, joys and sorrows; driven to discover beauty in people and things around us and to express it in a way that helps others see that beauty; very charming

Shadow: turns gift for lyricism into negative or destructive tool; supports military aggression or genocide.

Employment: author, artist, writer, teacher, alternative health, homeopath, massage and well-being, chiropractor

Priest
facilitates the making of spiritual vows and commitments to divine authority; rituals and ordination serve as a vehicle or spiritual channel of energy for others; accepts profound spiritual responsibilities; teaches by example

Shadow: inability to live according to teachings, especially morally; controls populace and interferes in politics for personal gain; misuses people's trust to satisfy sexual needs; glutton; hypocrite; deceiver; controls for personal gain; interferes in politics

Employment: priest, teacher, counselor, advocacy

Prince
a ruler-in-training who is in service to the people he will rule; generous; charming; lives by example; enjoys finer things in life; helpful to others; has a fun side; romantic; fights for what he believes; honorable; compassionate; dedicated to serving the greater good; integrity; ambitious; driven; natural leader; assertive; loves to make people laugh; very social; optimistic

Shadow: great feelings of entitlement; an heir apparent who uses his position solely for continuing an evil that already exists; will adopt all negative characteristics of the king; uses a ruler's shadow to advance his career and self-interest with little to no regard for the needs of others; arrogant; demanding; perfectionist; dominant

Employment: finance, corporate ownership, investments, entrepreneur

Prostitute

holds lessons in integrity; learns honesty with the self; has talents, ideas and other expression of the self; is able to birth and refine self-esteem and self-respect; learns to take care of the body; sensual; in-tune with the physical; allows energy to help with love and success within self-integrity; adaptable with change; healthy expression of the self; clear on values; aligns thoughts, words and actions

Shadow: has controlling interest in another person, as in selling one's own power; throws others under the bus (figuratively); fear of survival; dishonesty; self-imprisonment; allows people to use and drain energy, time, emotion and dignity; often takes unwanted jobs; disregards principles and health; sacrifices happiness for financial security

Employment: painter, writer, coaching, counseling, actor, publishing

Queen

leader; promotes power and authority in all women; astonishing ability to manage others from the safety of her home; promotes freedom, creativity and learning; wise; kind; loving; supportive; gentle yet powerful; magnetic aura

Shadow: prone to hysteria and dark powers, influences or plots; arrogance and defensiveness; aggressive and destructive patterns of behavior, particularly when she perceives her authority or capacity to maintain control over the court is being challenged; cold indifference to genuine needs of others (material or emotional); may not have a trustworthy support system; perfectionist

Employment: writer, artist, healer, psychologist, health and wellness, musician, research, yoga, dancer, psychic reader, business manager, politics

Rebel

key component of all human growth and development; powerful aid in helping to break out of old ways; helps others see past preconceptions in their fields of professional or creative endeavors; seeks out appropriate spiritual paths; gently empowers change using traditional and tribal approaches; creative; creates change slowly and at the right time

Shadow: rejects legitimate authority if it's difficult or unpleasant; evaluates rebellious impulses; difficult to follow rules; loss of trust and respect from others

Employment: vehicle sales, edgy clothing companies, activism, dance, politics inventions, technology

Rescuer

assists when needed and withdraws when done; provides an infusion of strength and support to help others survive difficult situations and crises; possesses stamina and inner knowledge to maneuver through themselves (more common in women); healing and empowering is essential; more common among women

Shadow: surfaces through a romantic connection in which one party seeks to establish an intimate bond by lending emotional support along with a hidden agenda that assumes the rescued party will return the Rescuer's romantic feelings; must hold someone in need of being rescued, lest they lose significance; burnout; treating the needs of others as more important; feels guilt if not assisting; feels deeply rejected if assistance is refused

Employment: civil servant, firefighter, healer; psychotherapist, massage therapist, doctor, veterinarian, teacher, psychologist

Saboteur

Make this archetype an ally, as it will alert you to situations where you are in danger of being sabotaged or sabotaging yourself; hears and heeds internal warnings; does not repeat past mistakes; self-acceptance, development and love; positively shaped by insight; has learned through trial and error

Shadow: self-destructive behavior or a desire to undermine others if warning signs are ignored; fears and issues related to low self-esteem cause them to make choices that block empowerment and success; resists healthy relationships; self doubt and distrust; victim; procrastinator; micromanages; overschedules

Employment: painter, writer, coaching, counseling, actor, publishing, psychologist

Sage
dominion over the mind; sees with clarity and vision; inspires people to gain knowledge, better life strategies and to achieve goals; great introspection for thinking on deep levels; combination of Hero, Explorer and Warrior archetypes; prepared to face life challenges; great imagination and innovation; relinquishes control and is adaptable; balance of heart and mind, thoughts and feelings, will and desire; wise without ego; positive; progressive

> *Shadow*: thinks too much rather than acts; great at starting things but not finishing them; obstinate, opinionated and impossible to reason with; lacks patience with those not their equal; too much control will undermine reaching their goals

Employment: education, coaching, career counseling, teaching, science, detective, philosopher

Samaritan
makes sacrifices for those least likely to get help (for example, stopping to give a stranger direction even if they are in a hurry); scribe; seeker; learns to choose carefully when helping to minimize hurt to someone or something else; selflessness; kindness; generosity; dedication; flashes of brilliance

> *Shadow*: helps one person or group to the detriment of another; similar to the Martyr; self-importance

Employment: storyteller, teacher, ghostwriter, social services, advocacy

Scribe

copies existing works in lieu of creating new ones; records existing knowledge and information of the day for the joy of sharing without personal gain; strong curiosity

> *Shadow*: alters facts; plagiarizes or sells information that belongs to others;

Employment: copyist, secretary, accountant, journalist, investigator, internet researching, transcribing, medical insurance coding, data entry, clerical, maintenance technician, computer technology, advanced algorithms

Seeker

searches on a path that may begin with earthly curiosity, but has at its core the search for God and/or enlightenment; searches for wisdom and truth wherever it can be found; learns to work with others as a team; searches for solutions; seeks to reinvent; wants to have deep understandings; pursues wisdom, knowledge and truth; desires enlightenment

> *Shadow*: infatuated with the trappings of a certain practice or guru; low self-esteem while empowering others; wants to perform their way; gets bored and frustrated easily; continually reinventing themselves, their products, organizations and services; too many projects at once; restless; looks outside of self; obsession

Employment: entrepreneur, creativity, editor, research

Servant

simultaneously in service to self and others; engages aspects of the psyche that call us to make ourselves available to others for the benefit and enhancement of their lives; very reliable; selflessness; compassion; dedicated to service; takes care of self first; develops self-esteem and boundaries

Shadow: consumed by needs of others and loses focus of the value of one's own life; makes choices that serve their highest potential; can neglect their own needs; must have acknowledgement and praise from others; burnout; gullible and naïve; difficulty setting boundaries; avoids conflict; unhealthy and abusive relationships; low self-esteem; insecure

Employment: teaching, nursing, social work, spiritual work

Shape-Shifter
ability to change appearances for a variety of reasons; navigates through different levels of consciousness, dream and waking states, and the astral plane; more flexible than the Trickster because the Shape-Shifter is not tied to a specific goal

Shadow: emphasizes instability, fickleness and lack of conviction; backstabber; revenge; struggle with self-definition; fact changing; big physical makeovers; changes changes; unpredictable

Employment: working with animals, dream analysis, sales, politics, actor

Slave
willing to do what needs to be done while setting bound-

aries; increases freedom; empathic; reclaims joy of serving; greater connection to humanity; greater purpose and meaning to life; can be clever; solves problems quickly

> *Shadow*: complete absence of power of choice and self-authority; lacks willpower for personal change; burnout; guilt; low self-esteem; victim thinking; Divine, cult and religious slave; easily manipulated like puppets; accepts scarcity and lack; disempowered; depressed; slave to their own ego

Employment: military, maid, shaman, ministry

Storyteller
relays wisdom and foolishness, mistakes and successes, facts and fiction, and tales of love and the impossible with balance; connects others with the inner self; able to use the voice effectively: communicates not just facts, but also a metaphoric learning or experience; has a deep connection to the human soul

> *Shadow*: liars in the extreme and exaggerators in the moderate; misuses the skill of storytelling to his own advantage; conceals truth; attention seeking

Employment: narrator, voiceovers, author, storyteller, teacher

Student
pattern of constant learning; openness to absorbing new information as an essential part of one's well-being; absence

of mastery of one subject, but continually pursues intellectual/spiritual development; curious

> *Shadow*: manifests in tandem with the shadow Teacher or Mentor, avidly learning the tools of the wrong trade or misusing the knowledge learned; also manifests as the eternal Student who never embarks on a life path; not ready or has not learned enough to advance his/her dreams

Employment: apprentice, secretary, playground attendant, department and grocery store worker

Thief

eventually gains self-respect; prods others to generate power from within; harsh self-development that leads to striving for dreams; strategic mind; learns there is greater power within; recognizes liars easily; earns skills for honest living; creative mind; has a sensitive sixth sense

> *Shadow*: swindler; con artist; pickpocket; burglar; rationalizes deeds for self and others; plagiarist; steals affection; feels inadequate and deprived; feels too intelligent to get caught; emotionally and intellectually compromised; untrustworthy; surrounded by like-minded individuals; dependent on others for financial support

Employment: security, police, detective, investigator, technology

Trickster

key figure in human drama; plays dubious jokes or tricks

without harming others; makes fun within boundaries; laughs at self when made fun of; the Creator's helper or messenger; great ally for presenting alternatives; liberates and transcends convention; non-conformist; creates realities of time and illusion; highly intelligent; crafty; seeks new ideas and experiences; brings new knowledge and wisdom

> *Shadow*: unsavory or duplicitous behavior; can have a dual personality; can camouflage as a demigod in religious circles; stuffy and distrustful; great insecurities of self; needs attention; scammer; creates chaos and mischief; sadistic; manipulative; cheating; master of disguise; tests people; destructive

Employment: magician, alchemist, clown, tactical jobs, escape artistry

Virgin

associated with purity and applied primarily to young girls; at a beginning point of creation; brings forth virgin ideas; monks and nuns channel sexual energy rather than repress it; hears the inner voice; cleanliness; pure heart; magnetic personality; curious; strong morals and ethics; analytical

> *Shadow*: prudish disgust with, or fear of, genuine sexuality; resists sex not to save energy, but because it seems inherently repellent; denies essential aspects of herself; represses sexual energy; manipulative; sacrificial power; prudish; passive; denial of self-aspects; overly innocent; reclusive; shy and introverted; overly sensitive and emo-

tional; avoids conflict; feels entitled; compares to others in a sense of superiority

Employment: jobs of service, religion

Visionary
imagines possibilities beyond the scope of individual life that benefit all of society; brings into view what could be inevitable if certain choices are made or have been made; enterprising; enjoys working with others

Shadow: willingness to sell one's visionary abilities to the highest bidder or to alter one's vision to make it more acceptable to society; tainted visions may lead entire societies into murderous or destructive rampages, allowing a Destroyer (Hitler-like) to supersede the Visionary:

Employment: artist, actor, filmmaker, journalist, writer, director, fashion designer, consultant, counselor, advocate, teacher, healer; music, dance, human resources, religion, career counselor, medicine, science

Warrior
represents physical strength and the ability to protect, defend and fight for one's rights; linked to invincibility and loyalty; energy is erotic for the male, representing the height of virility and physical power and toughness of will and spirit; being unbreakable and fighting to the death are associated with the passage from boyhood to manhood; feeds fantasies of independence and the power to defend ourselves and to right wrongs; stands up to injustice and holds off forces of evil single-handedly; women exhibit loyalty to family and tribe,

nurturing their young and transmitting lessons of power and self-defense; a spiritual warrior makes use of virtues of heroism and self-sacrifice to conquer the ego and gain control of inner lives; courageous; overcomes obstacles

> *Shadow*: hired killer who sells his power on the open market, often with complete disregard to the buyer's cause; assassin; can be truly evil, self-interested killers and thieves who embody our worst nightmares of lawlessness and unchecked male dominance; distorts or abandons ethical principles and decency in favor of risk and pain; indifferent to others; women may sacrifice body parts to facilitate warfare; vengefulness; sadism

Employment: military, police, medicine, firefighter, entrepreneur

Index

D

E

G

H

I

J

K

L

M

N

O

P

Q

R

S

T

U

V

W

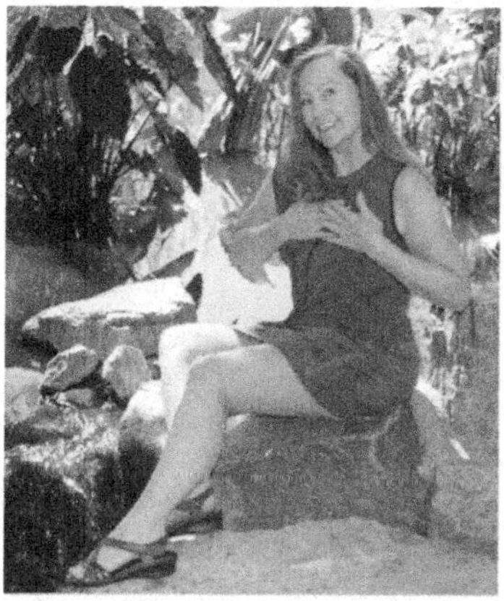

Connect with the Author

Sherry Bainbridge PhD, is a holistic health doctor, hypnotherapist, medical/spiritual intuitive, Reiki master and speaker. Her desire is to help others thrive regardless of the chaos around us.

Connect with Sherry through her website at:

holisticcollaboration.com

HOLISTIC COLLABORATION • BODY & SOUL NUTRITION •

Made in United States
North Haven, CT
10 November 2026

22088878R00192